RT
71
.C675
2000

D1279599

WITHDRAWN

JACKSON LIBRARY
LANDER UNIVERSITY
GREENWOOD, SC 29649

MC... N J. ...ONT

Springer Series on the Teaching of Nursing

Diane O. McGivern, RN, PhD, FAAN, Series Editor
New York University Division of Nursing

Advisory Board: *Ellen Baer, PhD, RN, FAAN; Carla Mariano, EdD, RN; Janet A. Rodgers, PhD, RN, FAAN; Alice Adam Young, PhD, RN*

Peggy Sherblom Matteson, PhD, RNC is an Associate Professor in the School of Nursing, Bouve College of Health Sciences, Northeastern University, Boston, MA. Certified as a women's health nurse practitioner, Dr. Matteson's practice and research interests focus on the lived experiences of women. Since September 1991, as part of her teaching responsibilities, she has been educating undergraduate students in the provision of women's health and collaborating with residents and providers in the neighborhood of Codman Square in Dorchester, MA. In addition, she collaborates with graduate students as they delve into health issues, ethics, and policy or acquire the skills of collaboration in the provision of the primary care with women.

Dr. Matteson is an author and frequent consultant to schools developing community-based nursing education programs. In addition, Dr. Matteson served as core faculty for the American Association of Colleges of Nursing/Helene Fuld Trust Project, Curriculum and Faculty Development in Community-Based Care for Undergraduate Nursing Education and project consultant to the 130 participating schools.

Community-Based Nursing Education

Peggy S. Matteson, PhD, RNC
Editor

 ***Springer Series on the
Teaching of Nursing***

JACKSON LIBRARY
LANDER UNIVERSITY
GREENWOOD, SC 29649

Copyright © 2000 by Springer Publishing Company, Inc.

All rights reserved

No part of this publication may be reproduced, stored in a retrieval system, or transmitted in any form or by any means electronic, mechanical, photocopying, recording, or otherwise, without the prior permission of Springer Publishing Company Inc.

Springer Publishing Company, Inc.
536 Broadway
New York, NY 10012-3955

Acquisitions Editor: Ruth Chasek
Production Editor: Janice Stangel
Cover design by James Scotto-Lavino

99 00 01 02 03 / 5 4 3 2 1

Library of Congress Cataloging-in-Publication Data

Community-based nursing education : the experience of eight schools
    of nursing / Peggy S. Matteson, editor.
     p.   cm.
    Includes bibliographical references and index.
    ISBN 0-8261-1323-0 (hardcover)
      1. Community health nursing—Study and teaching—United States.
    2. Nursing—Study and teaching—United States.   I. Matteson, Peggy.
    [DNLM: 1. Education, Nursing—methods—United States.
    2. Community Health Nursing—United States.   3. Community-
    Institutional Relations—United States.   4. Schools, Nursing—United
    States. WY 18 C7355 200]
    RT71 .C675 2000
    610.73'71'173—dc21   99-059687

Printed in the United States of America

This book is dedicated to the nursing students and faculty of:
American International College; Cleveland State University;
College of New Rochelle; Hartwick College; Northeastern University;
University of Central Florida; University of Rhode Island;
and Winston-Salem State University who stepped away from
tradition and to all of our community partners
who allowed us into your neighborhoods, homes, and hearts.
Our lives and our practices have been enriched beyond expectations.

CONTENTS

List of Illustrations and Tables

CONTRIBUTORS

Ayesha Ali, MS, RN
Assistant Professor
Division of Nursing
American International College
Springfield, Massachusetts

Joan Arnold, PhD, RN
Associate Professor
School of Nursing
College of New Rochelle
New Rochelle, New York

Carol Hardin Boles, MS, RN
Director
University/Community Wellness
   Center
Winston-Salem State University
Winston-Salem, North Carolina

Marilyn Breuer, MS, RN
Assistant Professor
Division of Nursing
American International College
Springfield, Massachusetts

Deborah Godfrey Brown, MS, RN
Assistant Professor and Director of
   the Undergraduate Program
College of Nursing
University of Rhode Island
Kingston, Rhode Island

Margot De Sevo, PhD, RNC
Assistant Professor
School of Nursing
College of New Rochelle
New Rochelle, New York

Sharon D. Dettenrieder, RN, MSN
Asociate Professor of Nursing
Hartwick College
Oneonta, New York

Mary Alice Donius, EdD, RN
Associate Professor
School of Nursing
College of New Rochelle
New Rochelle, New York

Anne DuVal Frost, PhD, RN
Associate Professor
School of Nursing
College Of New Rochelle
New Rochelle, New York

Marylee Evans, MS, RN
Assistant Professor
College of Nursing
University of Rhode Island
Kingston, Rhode Island

Sylvia Ann Flack, EdD, RN
Director and Professor
Division of Health Sciences
Winston-Salem University
Winston-Salem, North Carolina

Jeanne-Marie E. Havener, MS, RNC
Assistant Professor of Nursing
Hartwick College
Oneonta, New York

Ermalynn Kiehl, PhD, ARNP
Assistant Professor
University of Central Florida
Orlando, Florida

Jeanne M. Leffers, PhD, RN
Assistant Professor
College of Nursing
University of Rhode Island
Kingston, Rhode Island

Margaret Ann Mahoney, PhD, RNC
Assistant Professor
School of Nursing
Bouve College of Health Sciences
Northeastern University
Boston, Massachusetts

Diane C. Martinez, Med, RN
Assistant Professor
College of Nursing
University of Rhode Island
Kingston, Rhode Island

Cheryl P. McCahon, PhD, RN
Director, Undergraduate Program
Associate Professor
Department of Nursing
Cleveland State University
Cleveland, Ohio

Sheila A. Niles, MSN, RNC
Director of Community Projects &
    Elder Health and Elder Care Plus
Visiting Nurse Association of
    Cleveland and;
Faculty
Case Western Reserve University
Cleveland State University
Cleveland, Ohio

Karen Rousseau, MS, RNC
Assistant Professor
Division of Nursing;
Coordinator of the RN to BSN
    Program
American International College
Springfield, Massachusetts

Marie Santiago, EdD, RNC
Associate Professor
School of Nursing
College of New Rochelle
New Rochelle, New York

Marie Truglio Londrigan, PhD, RNC
Faculty
University of Medicine and Dentistry
Newark, New Jersey

Geraldine Valencia-Go, PhD, RNC
Associate Professsor
School of Nursing
College of New Rochelle
New Rochelle, New York

Eileen Zungolo, EdD, RN
Dean and Professor
School of Nursing
Bouve College of Health Sciences
Northeastern University
Boston, Massachusetts

Preface

Peggy Matteson

In 1991, when we initiated our community-based nursing education program for the College of Nursing at Northeastern University in Boston, MA, we had a vision and a desire. With the persuasive and constant input of our community partners the program has created unique processes and practices for our nursing students that are successful educational experiences others continue to evolve toward success.

After several years, the faculty, administrators, and our community partners started to share their experiences in the professional literature and were invited to speak at professional programs and consult with other schools. Word of our collaborative activities also spread with the publication of a book, *Nursing in the Neighborhoods—The Northeastern University Model* (Matteson, 1995). A growing number of faculty started asking if they could come to Boston to see what we did. Having a steady flow of visitors in and out of our clinical sites would have proved too disruptive. Instead, with the assistance of our community partners, we developed a faculty development program, the Summer Institute on Nursing in the Neighborhoods, first held in 1996.

The Summer Institute guided participants from the general information, such as why we had changed our program, to the specific information that described in detail what we had done and how we did it. We included those things that had worked and those that hadn't as well as the things we were still trying to implement. We shared the joys and challenges of changing a whole curriculum as well as changing course content and clinical objectives. One day was spent out in a neighborhood clinical area so that the visiting faculty, now turned students, could engage in the initial steps of orientation to a neighborhood, interacting with and learning from the providers and residents of a neighborhood.

After faculty returned to their schools, we often heard from them as they tried to adapt what they had learned into their own academic and neighborhood communities. All but two of the examples within this book are provided by participants in one of the Institutes. The exceptions are "Vision on 22nd Street" and "The Violence Intervention and Prevention Program (VIP)." "Vision of 22nd Street" contributes a successful educational endeavor that is unique. "The Violence Intervention and Prevention Program" is an example of a service learning project within a community-based nursing education program. The VIP program allows a small number of undergraduate and graduate students to provide a specific range of services to specific neighborhoods as part of their clinical education and cooperative education work experience or through independent study.

Just as each neighborhood is unique so must be every community-based nursing education program. Each of these programs demonstrates a unique way in which the principles of community-based education (a partnership between academia and community through which clinical services emerge from the capacities of the community and the nursing program in response to needs identified by the community) may be implemented either in a portion of or across the curriculum. The book is a testimony to creative and innovative projects that emerge when creative faculty and community partners work together. We continue to learn from each other as we move the process of nursing education forward, educating the nurses of the future.

1

Preparing Nurses For The Future

Peggy Matteson

Interest and excitement in the community-based education paradigm has grown rapidly during the last five years. Many nursing programs are now trying to determine how they might integrate the concept of partnering with neighborhoods for the benefit of both the students and the residents.

COMMUNITY-BASED EDUCATIONAL PEDAGOGY

Community-based education is an educational pedagogy that requires a partnership between at least two communities: academia and a neighborhood. It is a method of teaching that embraces and values the knowledge and skills of all participants (faculty, students, providers, and residents). It enables participants to work collaboratively to improve the health of individuals, groups, and the neighborhood as a whole while educating faculty and students in the realities of patient or client lives.

Community-based education enables students to learn to care for people no matter where they are. The nature of the pedagogy requires different teaching strategies and unconventional settings. To assist the students in the process of learning from multiple people in new arenas we must move from a role of "sage on the stage" to that of facilitator and "guide on the side." In addition, as part of a partnership, the role of "guide" will also be assumed by other providers and the potential recipients of care. The students become colleagues in care.

The curriculum content for community-based education includes: professional values; the core competencies of critical thinking, communication, assessment and technical skills; the core knowledge of nursing health promotion, risk reduction and disease prevention; illness and disease management; information and health care technologies; ethics; human diversity; global health care; health care systems; and policy development; and role development as a health care designer, manager, and coordinator (AACN, 1998). [Refer to Table 1-1.]

A community-based educational program does not automatically negate the assignment of students to clinical rotations within institutions. Institutions, such as hospitals and long-term care facilities, are located to serve communities and are a part of the continuum of nursing care provided to residents. It does, however, improve the care students and then graduates provide in acute care settings. Their partnering with neighborhood residents provides them with a more realistic understanding of the choices and compromises that occur in the daily lives of individuals and their families.

A community is a social group determined by geographical boundaries and/or common values and interests. The people within a community interrelate within a particular social structure, exhibit and create norms and values, and establish social institutions that fulfill the functions of the community (World Health Organization, 1978). This WHO definition of community contains the components we commonly associate with the denotation of a neighborhood.

To emphasis that the concept of community-based education is distinct from community nursing, the title *Teaching Nursing in the Neighborhoods—The Northeastern University Model* was selected for our first book. The term neighborhood implies a small, more homogeneous grouping of people than does the area and number of people often encompassed within a community. In fact, communities are often made up of many neighborhoods, each with different views and agendas. For community-based education to be successful, we must pay attention to both the self-selecting identification as being from a neighborhood as well as the broader understanding of what it means to be part of a community.

NURSING PRACTICE ROLES

Due to similarity in terms and the location of practice experiences, there is sometimes confusion between the educational pedagogy and the practice roles of nurses. The educational experiences in a community-based program may appear to be those that are "generally associated with community nursing which encompass a variety of services that emerge from the

TABLE 1-1 Differentiating between the art of teaching, the content taught, and the practice areas for application of knowledge

Pedagogy	Curriculum/Course Content	Role/Practice Area
Community-Based Nursing Education • Involves those educational experiences generally associated with community nursing which encompass a variety of services that emerge from the needs and capacities of both the community and educational entities. • Requires an ongoing and true partnership between education and the community. • Each community becomes a unique context for education.	(Determined by mission statement of institution, requirements of accrediting body, state Board of Registration, goals of the curriculum, goals and objectives of the course, instructors' areas or interest and expertise, and students' interests and potential career choices) *Essentials of Baccalaureate Education for Professional Nursing Practice:* • Liberal education integrated with nursing education • Professional values: altruism, autonomy, human dignity, integrity, and social justice. • Core competencies: critical thinking, communication, assessment, and technical skills.	We are preparing people to respond as professional nurses in a variety of roles, with diverse populations in variant places, such as: • acute care nursing • addictions nursing • ambulatory care • college health nursing • community health nursing • correctional facilities nursing • diabetes nursing • genetics nursing • gerontological nursing • health care lobbyist • home health nursing

(continued)

3

TABLE 1-1 (*continued*)

Pedagogy	Curriculum/Course Content	Role/Practice Area
	• Core knowledge: health promotion, risk reduction and disease prevention; illness and disease management; information and health care technologies; ethics, human diversity, global health care, health care systems and health care policy. • Role development: provider of care, designer/manager/coordinator of care, and contributing member of a profession. (AACN,1998)	• maternal child nursing • neonatal nursing • nursing administration • nursing informatics • obstetric nursing • oncology nursing • parish nursing • pediatric nursing • perinatal nursing • psychiatric-mental health • respiratory nursing • rehabilitation nursing • school nursing • women's health nursing, and • other areas yet to be developed.

needs of the community, and are characterized by interdisciplinary effort" (NLN, 1997). To be clear in our discussion we must discern the definitions of commonly used terms. The following definitions of nursing practice roles have been derived from the work of the organizations providing leadership in this arena.

"Public health nursing synthesizes the body of knowledge from the public health sciences and professional nursing theories for the purpose of improving the health of the entire community. This goal lies at the heart of primary prevention and health promotion and is the foundation for public health nursing practice. . . ." (APHA, 1981, p. 10).

"Community health nursing practice promotes and preserves the health of populations by integrating the skills and knowledge relevant to both nursing and public health" (ANA, 1986, p. 1). The dominant responsibility of the community health nurse is to the population as a whole, the public's health. When care is given to individuals, families, and groups, the nurse determines which clients to serve as determined by the assessment of the needs of the population. The terms community nursing and public health nursing were defined as synonymous (ANA, 1986).

In 1990, the Task Force on Community Health Nursing Education, Association of Community Health Nursing Educators (ACHNE) agreed that the terminology of community health nursing and public health nursing are synonymous. The provision of nursing service is to the community of people as a whole based on the needs of the whole. Individuals or families receive care only when they are part of the group at risk being cared for by the nurse.

The health care of the aggregates is improved not only by providing nursing care but also through political activity aimed at improving social and environmental conditions. Public health nurses promote health and prevent disease for entire population groups by working with others providers of care to plan, develop, and support systems and programs in the community to prevent problems and provide access to care (APHA, 1996, pp. 1, 2).

IMPLEMENTING COMMUNITY-BASED NURSING EDUCATION

Community-based nursing education brings together three components: the members of the university (students and faculty), the providers in the community, and the members of the community. They work together to create and implement the educational program. The components of a community-based nursing education program are:

- An ongoing and true partnership in which the voices of the community are heard
- Interventicns developed in response to the needs identified by the community
- Interventions emerging from the capacities of the community and the nursing program

The process of developing and implementing a program of community-based education is unique within each school. Our ongoing work, however, with schools changing to community-based education has revealed the identification of common concerns. These are:

- How to reach agreement with all the participants on a vision
- The work of changing the curriculum yet again
- The process of developing a partnership with a neighborhood
- How to meet the actual or perceived learning needs of the students
- How to evaluate the students' work
- The success of the students on the N-CLEX examination
- The employment of graduates

Information and guidance from those that have been successful will help answer your questions and move your quest for community-based nursing education forward.

WHY MOVE TO COMMUNITY-BASED EDUCATION?

The health care system is moving from an array of disconnected agencies to integrated systems. Nursing practice is increasingly focused on health promotion/disease prevention. This occurs where people live, work, and play. Competence in community-based practice therefore requires clinical learning opportunities beyond the usual direct practice-type designed for individuals seeking care (AACN, 1999).

The pedagogy of community-based nursing education provides the means for preparing the nurses of the future. It requires partnerships with other disciplines and with community members to develop effective interventions for individual, groups, and the neighborhood.

"There is no such thing as a neutral educational process. Education either functions as an instrument to bring the younger generation into the present system and bring about conformity to it, or it becomes the practice of freedom, as men and women deal critically and creatively with reality and discover how to participate in the transformation of their world." R. Schaull

Are you participating in the education of nurses who will conform to the present system or are you educating nurses who will discover and participate in the future of nursing care? This book offers examples of how a variety of schools have creatively addressed the issue of preparing nurses to transform their world. It provides encouragement to move forward, with each school finding its own unique way based on the assets and requirements of the partners involved.

REFERENCES

American Nurses Association (ANA). (1986). *Standards of Community Health Nursing Practice.* (ANA Pub. No. CH-2) Washington, DC: Author.

American Association of Colleges of Nursing (AACN). (1998). *The Essentials of Baccalaureate Education for Professional Nursing Practice.* Washington, DC: Author.

American Association of Colleges of Nursing (AACN). (1999). *Essential Clinical Resources for Nursing's Academic Mission.* Washington, DC: Author.

American Public Health Association (APHA). (1981). *The definition and role of public health nursing practice in the delivery of health care: A statement of the public health nursing section.* Washington, DC: Author.

American Public Health Association, Public Health Nursing Section (APHA). (1996). *The definition and role of public health nursing—A statement of the Public Health Nursing Section.* Washington, DC: Author.

Association of Community Health Nursing Educators, Task Force on Basic Community Health Nursing Education (ACHNE). (1990). *Essentials of baccalaureate nursing education for entry level community health nursing practice.* Louisville, KY: Author.

National League of Nursing. (1997). *Visions II community-based nursing education project. Final Report.* New York: Author.

Schaull, R. (1989) Foreward in *Pedagogy of the oppressed* by P. Freire, New York: Continuum.

World Health Organization. *Alma-Ata 1978-Primary Health Care: Report of the International Conference on Primary Health Care, Alma-Ata, USSR.* Geneva, Switzerland: Author.

2

Changing Nursing Education

Eileen Zungolo

The 1990s have witnessed a dramatic shift in the locus and orientation of nursing education. While once the hospital was Mecca for the education of future nurses, educators are looking beyond that venue and far beyond the parameters of traditional extra-institutional sites. Essentially, nursing education, especially baccalaureate nursing-education, has moved from the tertiary setting to a community-based approach. The impact on the work of the National League for Nursing, in the "Curriculum Revolution" and the publications related to that effort has been important to this evolutionary process. Of equal importance has been the pioneering work of the W. K. Kellogg Foundation in its efforts to improve health care in the United States and other countries through the enhancement of health professions education.

W. K. KELLOGG COMMUNITY PARTNERSHIP INITIATIVE

In 1989, the Kellogg Foundation launched the Community Partnerships Initiative which had as its central purpose the development of health professionals for the primary care arena. Building on its strong history in this area, the Foundation proposed a comprehensive enterprise in which, at a minimum, medical and nursing students would learn together in community-based settings. A central theme of this proposal, however, was the partnership building aspect which fostered engaging members of the consumer community, health care recipients, and community activists in the formulation of a new perspective on the education of health professionals. In addition to the sweeping ambition of the initiative, the leaders, Dr. Ronald Richards and Dr. Helen Grace, designed a creative approach to the proposal development that maximized the interaction of all the participants. This led to the creation of a cadre of experts in health professions education for primary care.

In the Fall of 1989, the initial RFP which required a minimum of a medical school and a nursing school led to a strong response from educators in the field. Of the 127 medical schools at the time, all but 10 partnered with a nursing education program and responded with a letter of intent. The initial screening by the W. K, Kellogg Foundation produced 15 semi-finalist collaborating groups. These institutions, and the evolving partnerships they represented, then participated in a year-long planning process in which teams from the 15 groups met on four separate occasions for a week at a time. The "networking" meetings were important on a number of levels to the participants and the donors. Essentially, it was during these sessions that the various groups began to develop a "vision," an idea, a concept about community partnerships in health professions education, and began to understand what community-based education would and could entail within the context of the rapidly changing health services milieu.

Although this learning was important, of critical value was getting to know the other teams, the nature of their evolving projects, and how we could learn from each other and support each other. There were interesting discoveries about one's self as well. The 15 teams were essentially competitors for the same financial award. Not all of us would be chosen as the recipients of the $6 million grants. As a result, there was some occasional discussion about the relative value of withholding information from other teams, as concern that concepts and approaches would be used by others, limiting the "creativity" of one project over another. Most of the participants, however, also developed genuine friendships, many of which continue to exist some 10 years later. At the same time, and so important to the long-term quality of the project, authentic and passionate commitment to the notion of community partnerships and primary care was formed and shared, along with the ideas.

The various teams were not without the competitive edge either, but invariably spiced with good humor. For example, it was well known to all participants that there would be 6 or maybe 7 of the 15 projects funded at the $6 million dollar level. By the sixth month of the planning year the humor and adventure of the group had led to a "pool" in which funds were wagered on who would be the "final 6." This "pool" changed regularly as the nature of the partnerships began to unfold and as the curriculum and programmatic implications became clearer. None of these high-level gamblers (maximum bet $2) were 100% right when the final awards were made, but many had accurately guessed 5 of the final 6. The awards went to: the University of Hawaii, a partnership in Texas between the University of Texas at El Paso and Texas Tech; East Tennessee University; a partnership in Atlanta with Morehead University, Emory University, and Georgia State University; a partnership in West Virginia between all the state schools and Marshall University; Michigan State University; and the Boston partnership of the Center for Community Health, Education, Research, and Service (better known as CCHERS).

CENTER FOR COMMUNITY HEALTH, EDUCATION, RESEARCH AND SERVICE (CCHERS)

Located in Boston, this unique partnership was composed of Boston University School of Medicine, Northeastern University College of Nursing, the City of Boston's Department of Health and Hospitals, and originally four neighborhood health centers. (In 1991 this number was expanded to 10 neighborhood partners.)

Originally, it was thought that the administrative office of CCHERS, ably led by Executive Director Dr. Patricia Mcguire Meservey from the College of Nursing, would function as the "hub of the wheel," with the neighborhoods and the academic partners functioning as the spokes. As time went on, however, it became apparent that each of the neighborhood health centers functioned as a neighborhood "hub" for student learning experiences, with health promotion activities extending throughout the multiple neighborhoods of Boston.

COLLEGE OF NURSING PARTNERS WITH NEIGHBORHOODS

After review of the undergraduate program, the College of Nursing determined that many of the elements of the program were too traditional. With the development of the partnership, the faculty began a joint exploration of ways in which the curriculum could be modified to achieve a more community-based orientation. The college was fortunate at that time to have among its members some very talented and forward-thinking faculty and administrators. A team from within the college was formed and developed some strong support strategies, as we created ways to address the concerns and hesitation many of the faculty experienced when thinking about abandoning many of our traditional, hospital-based methods of teaching nursing and developing a community-based undergraduate program.

The partners in the community were of considerable assistance to us and, in many respects, provided the traditional program planners with a new window through which to view the planning phases. For example, the educators began to think about various learning experiences that might be available to our students in the community and to address those courses in which community-based experiences made "sense." Our partners, on the other hand, advocated that the students have experiences in the community as part of **all** their courses. The faculty considered many ways in which the students could be "rotated" through the various neighborhoods, while our partners advocated for consistent placement of the students in one neighborhood. In almost all these discussions our experience has demonstrated that the "community members," whether residents, community health center employees, or health practitioners, were right! In fact, I remain convinced that many of the most successful and innovative ideas for the implementation of our community-based curriculum came from the inspired commitment of the community.

Through multiple processes and strategies, the curriculum of the undergraduate program was changed early in 1991, and the decision was made to create a transition plan which would enable the community-based approach to be implemented at once. In addition to the belief that community-based education was the wave of the future and would prepare out students better, we did not want to wait five years prior to having the full undergraduate program in place. Carole Shea, PhD, RN, FAAN, then Associate Dean of Academic Affairs for the College of Nursing, did an excellent job designing the implementation plan.

The initial faculty members who spearheaded the community-based instruction were nurse practitioner faculty committed to the role of primary care in health promotion, experienced teachers, and expert in extra institutional health care settings. These individuals, especially Barbara Kelley, Mary Ann Gauthier, Peggy Matteson and Margaret Mahoney, brought their enthusiasm, creativity, and exceptional problem-solving capacity to the task. While in the beginning some things did not work as expected, the community-based curriculum began to experience success and become a reality. As the program continues to evolve, we build on our successes, learn from our partners, and implement new experiences for students.

CONTINUED EVOLUTION OF COMMUNITY-BASED NURSING EDUCATION

Much has happened in the intervening years since we started in 1991 to give the community-based curriculum significant credibility within nursing education. Now, most, if not all, nursing programs have some elements of their curriculum located in a community setting. There are many issues within this approach, however, which have not been addressed and many others which have emerged over the years. There are, unfortunately, many interpretations of community-based education, some of which paint an erroneous picture of the nature of this learning. Other issues emerge from the efforts of faculty to enter the community and begin the process. An experience I had in the recent past has provided some insights into these dimensions that may provide a viewing glass to the programs that are described in subsequent chapters.

NLN VISIONS II PROJECT

In 1993, the president of the National League for Nursing, Dr. Carol Lindeman, PhD, RN, FAAN, spearheaded the development of the Visions Project. She was successful in obtaining funds from the W. K. Kellogg Foundation to assist nurse educators in the transition to community-based nursing education. The Visions II Project of 1995 built on previous work and was specifically designed to assess the nature and extent of barriers to community-based nursing education as well as develop models for implementation. In Phase II, the NLN selected four constituents (Minnesota, Texas, Hawaii, and Massachusetts/Rhode Island [MARILN]) to serve as pilot projects.

The opportunity to serve as the Project Director for the MA/RI constituent league was a unique privilege on a number of fronts. It had always been a lament of ours at Northeastern that we had not kept journals of the processes that emerged during our community partnership development. To have such a record of personal observations during the time of upheaval and change could have provided insight into many of the dimensions of adjustment, compromise, and learning that we all experienced.

Working with the nurse educators of the constituent league offered the promise of viewing the process that people use when undertaking such a serious change. While unable to utilize vigorous qualitative research methods, I did have the chance to note a number of similarities in the participants of the Vision II Project and the faculty at Northeastern as we dealt with change.

Another area of keen interest relates to the systematic identification of the barriers to community-based nursing education. While we had long heard many arguments against the move to the community and the problems inherent in that, there had been no chance to systematically delineate these variables. Although community-based education continues its expansion, we continue to hear the same arguments advanced against it. During the MARILN Visions II Project, some possible barriers were identified by participants. I will examine the impact the perceived barriers have on emerging practices in nursing education.

CLINICAL DIMENSIONS OF NURSING EDUCATION

Nursing education has long based its approach to student learning on the assignment and management of patients with deviations from health which were most commonly treated in an acute care setting. Curriculum content has been organized and based in the medical model and geography of the traditional hospital. Even courses designed to enable students to work in Visiting Nurse Services and Home Health have relied heavily on an acute care model of practice. Although the last 20 years witness the use of many different titles for nursing courses, most approaches have remained relatively constant. Curriculum development in nursing has been somewhat static with considerable effort expanded to make internal modifications in the way in which curriculum is organized. The net result, however, infrequently yielded insignificant change in focus, orientation, or delivery.

THE HEALTH CARE ENVIRONMENT

In the present shifting health care milieu of the 1990s organized nursing has taken a leadership position which has included developing recommendations for new approaches to health care and working extensively with federal and national groups to examine current practices and make recommendations for change. Examples of these efforts abound in *Nursing's Agenda for Health Care Reform* (ANA, 1991), the *NLN Position Paper on Nursing Education* (NLN, 1993), the *Vision of Baccalaureate and Graduate Nursing Education: The next decade* (AACN, 1997), the *Essentials of Baccalaureate Education for Professional Nursing Practice* (AACN, 1998), and *Essential Clinical Resources for Nursing's Academic Mission* (AACN, 1999).

The Pew Commission's recommendations for revision of health professionals' education (1991) have been particularly influential in highlighting the need to refocus preparation toward primary care. All of these documents represent extensive analysis and have advocated a substantial investment in the education of health professionals who are as knowledgeable about the promotion of health and prevention of disease as they are about the management of deviations from health.

THE MASSACHUSETTS AND RHODE ISLAND AREA

Massachusetts and Rhode Island, and in particular Boston, have long been noted as having premiere sites for medical services. Influenced by an array of medical schools, New England has historically been very influential in the evolution of technology and discoveries that mark significant advances in medical practices. The era of managed care, however, has changed much of that and many of the most prestigious of academic health science centers and managed care organizations are rapidly losing money and are increasingly vulnerable to external factors which are not focused on quality control.

Nursing, too, has made outstanding contributions to the advancement of health services and education in the delivery of health services in the region. Nonetheless, it could be argued that the medical successes and technological progress in New England have, in some ways, held the advancement of nursing back and impeded the development of community-based nursing. With a few notable exceptions, nursing within New England and particularly the Commonwealth of Massachusetts has been a stepchild to medicine. Underappreciated and underpaid through most of their history, the nurses of the region have long experienced the paternalism that flows from the male medical hierarchy. Massachusetts is a state heavily dependent on the health care industry as an essential element of its economy. Medicine, perceived as an income generator, has dominated as a source of income, while nursing, perceived as a debit in the hospital accounting system, continues to struggle to maintain standards of care in quality staffing.

As managed care has increased its penetration within the Commonwealth, the balance of power in the health care industry is demonstrating some remarkable shifts and significant power struggles. The hospitals continue in a frenzy of mergers, coupled with an overall significant decrease in hospital capacity and patient care days. This has resulted in downsizing, with a shortage of nursing resources occurring in the acute care institutions.

With these events, community-based services are growing rapidly and exerting influence on the once omnipotent hospital administration-medical staff dyad. Hospital administrators recognize the need to partner with the community to ensure a revenue stream; they are branching out into the community and offering new services to maintain market share. The efficacy of primary care as a cost saving tool is gaining recognition, particularly within large managed care organizations.

In addition to the changes in the distribution of services, there are changes in the deployment of staff in health care arenas that have a strong impact on the nature of the nursing education and the quality of nursing education learning experiences. Funds formerly available to facilitate the educational process in institutions are drying up. As efforts to reward cost efficiencies increase, there is less impetus for staff to participate in student learning, leading to a decline in opportunities for students in clinical education. This impact of managed care, coupled with Medicare and Medicaid reform, threatens to seriously impact the funds available to engage in clinical learning and teaching, the historic heart of nursing education. Nursing within the region has struggled to find its voice in this medically dominated environment and has learned that in unity there is strength. As a result, the nursing community has made a strong commitment to work together in partnership.

MARILN VISIONS PROJECT

The long-term objective of the Massachusetts/Rhode Island League of Nursing Visions Project (MARILN) was to foster a consumer-driven, community-based system of health professions education to meet the primary care needs of citizens. In order to achieve this goal, the project aimed to explore the nature and extent of obstacles to community-based nursing education and to develop strategies to address these barriers. Within the MARILN approach we developed a strong Task Force highly representative of all areas of nursing education, practice and service as well as consumers.

Consensus Building

Five consensus building meetings were held over a one-year period throughout the two-state constituency with a total attendance of over 500 of whom almost 200 participants attended two or more meetings.

Most of the meetings included presentations by experts in community-based education, however, the heart of the meetings were small group break-out sessions. Within these small discussion groups, Task Force members were deployed to take notes and foster the recording of ideas. All notes were then used in a multistage process of analysis, tabulated, cross referenced, and summarized. Ideas, definitions, and barriers were all developed using this initial process and then discussed, summarized and outlined by the Task Force.

The Work of the Task Force

The initial meeting of the Task Force to plan the Consensus Building Meetings identified the difficulties that we could expect within the project as a whole. All members of this committee had very different ideas and opinions about the most elemental factors related to community-based education. This has been a consistent experience in working with various groups around the country, i.e., we lack a common frame of reference, including agreement on basic definitions.

Clarification of Terms

The first step had to be the development of a glossary. Since they are often used interchangeably, the terms to be defined were: community, community nursing, public health nursing, and community-based nursing education. During the first consensus building meeting, over 200 participants worked in 15 small groups to develop the components included in the definitions of the identified terms. The Task Force took the information for analysis and inclusion in development of the definitions through the consensus building process.

It is interesting to note that, although two of the following definitions are established definitions from existing professional groups, the process to arrive at these definitions was consistent with the processes used throughout the project to arrive at consensus.

Glossary

COMMUNITY

Where individuals and groups live, work, and interact, including local and global geographic areas.

COMMUNITY HEALTH NURSING

Nursing practice which promotes and preserves the health of populations by integrating the skills and knowledge relevant to both nursing and public health. The practice is comprehensive and general, and is not limited to a particular age or diagnostic group; it is continual, and is not limited to episodic care. While community health nursing practice includes nursing directed to individuals, families, and groups, the dominant responsibility is to the population as a whole. (ANA, 1986)

PUBLIC HEALTH

Focuses on health promotion and disease prevention for global populations under governmental control. Factors include, but are not inclusive of, public safety, inspections, investigations, epidemiology, environmental concerns, and surveillance.

Public Health Nursing

Synthesizes the body of knowledge from the public health sciences and professional nursing theories for the purpose of improving the health of the entire community. This goal lies at the heart of the primary prevention and health promotion and is the foundation for public health nursing practice. To accomplish this goal, public health nurses work with groups, families, and individuals as well as in multidisciplinary teams and programs. Identifying the subgroups (aggregates) within the population which are at high risk of illness, disability, or premature death and directing resources toward these groups is the most effective approach for accomplishing the goal of public health nursing (APHA, 1981).

Exactly what community-based nursing education is and is not resides at the heart of this entire process of defining terms. Achieving consensus within nursing education about this definition remains a critical issue as we strive to develop clarity and a consistent frame of reference.

Community-based Nursing Education

Those educational experiences generally associated with community nursing which encompass a variety of services that emerge from the needs of the community and are characterized by interdisciplinary effort. Community-based nursing education requires a partnership between education and the community.

COMPONENTS OF COMMUNITY-BASED NURSING EDUCATION

There are several elements in the above definition that differentiate true community-based nursing education from clinical-oriented experiences that happen to occur in the community. Of primary importance here is the partnership between the education and community.

Our experience at Northeastern University with the communities of Boston consistently brought this aspect of the learning program home. When we became fixated on achieving a certain learning experience for our students because it emanated from the course objectives and not from community interest or commitment, the experience was short-lived and not successful. On the other hand, when experiences arose from the observed need of some element of the community, the experience flourished.

For example, on many occasions the faculty attempted programmatic ventures designed to strengthen our experiences with the healthy aged and achieved marginal success. When members of that group identified a need, however, a sustainable program was born. One of the faculty members, Mary Ann Gauthier, had a group of students who visited a senior citizen residence as part of a broadly based community assignment. During the course of one of these sessions, the faculty members observed a 90+- year-old woman looking out the window to a nearby athletic track which was part of the urban community center. The faculty member inquired, "What are you thinking about?" to which the advanced senior replied, " I was thinking how much I would love to walk on that track before I die." And thus began the senior walking group.

With the planning of a creative faculty member (Dr. Mary Ann Gauthier), a side remark was turned into a consistent activity for these old-sters. When students are in place at the facility, they join the walk and engage in reminiscence therapy with the residents and obtain comprehensive family and health histories. Of even more importance, a meaningful outlet for the elderly was found which is not only pleasant but also good for them. Simultaneously, the students develop new insights into the stamina and yearnings of the elderly, no matter how advanced in years they may be chronologically. The students also gain a consistent and long-term way to build enduring relationships with senior citizens that enhance student learning about the needs of this age group.

Long-Term Commitment of Educational Institution and Community

We, the nursing faculty at Northeastern University, have found that the secret to sustaining meaningful, long-term learning experiences for students is assuring a link between the community residents and the learners. As the participants develop strong bonds, the community is more open to the students and to establishing a long-term commitment to the concept of student learning.

This notion of long-term commitment is important from two perspectives. First, the relationship that needs to be built with the community requires that the educational institution champion the values of the community and commit to serve those on a consistent and responsive basis. Historically the communities of the United States, particularly in the urban arena, have been used by educational institutions for its goals, independent of the needs and desires of the community. In fact the establishment of the network of neighborhood health centers in Boston occurred to protect the community from the transit nature of interest from the health care establishments. Repeatedly, when the health care institutions or educational institutions had grants or wanted to undertake research in the urban setting, they would expect the community to participate, not just willingly, but gratefully! This form of usury, in addition to being unethical, led to the formation of distrust and avoidance on the part of the community. The community must trust the educational institution to be true to its word, to be responsive to its needs and to be forthright in the identification of limitations. The development of a trusting partnership can occur when committed community leaders who want the best for their residents are willing to work with committed educational institutions to achieve shared goals.

Second, the students need to develop a long-term relationship with the community. In the early days of our partnership, when the communities wanted the students to return to the same neighborhoods for their experiences, I initially saw only the nightmare of scheduling and planning such an approach would entail. Nevertheless, I saw that this was an important value of the community, hence, we agreed that the nursing students would be assigned to a "neighborhood" in their first clinical experience and return to that site with each subsequent course. This continuity component has developed as one of the strongest elements of the program. Not only do the students identify with the community, but also the community identifies with the individual student. Over the four-year period of clinical study the student will have had experiences in almost every dimension of the neighborhood: the schools; the neighborhood health center clinics; outreach programming; senior citizens day care programs and residences; neighborhood health programming; Visiting Nurse Associations; Home Health units; and, oh yes, hospitals! Hence, the culminating senior community assessment project is a comprehensive, historically full account of the evolution of a group of people living together sharing common goals, and sometimes, common health problems.

"Fit" Between Educational Institution and Community-Based Education

Another area of concern is that, too often, the nature and purpose of the community experience and its "fit" with the total program of learning has not been well thought out. All too often, schools and faculty are so eager to have diversity of learning experiences for their students that they are failing to engage with the community in a consistent approach.

Within the last two years I chaired a Program Evaluation Team for the National League for Nursing Accrediting Commission (NLNAC) in which the diversity of student learning experiences was touted by one and all to be a strength of the program. In discussion with students they boasted to me that their community-based program was so rich that they had never been to the same clinical setting twice! These students did not have community-based education, rather they had a scattered collection of "visits" to health care agencies located outside of a hospital. In the course of my discussion with these students, they were very limited in the ability to describe their learning. In fact, in response to specific questions focused on what they had learned, they were only able to describe how they got to the agency, superficial information about the services offered, and to whom they reported. They knew nothing about the community, its values, its culture, its major health concerns, its problem solving capacities, or how they as students could contribute to the community. In short, these collected experiences were in the community, but not of the community. Hence, the notion of partnership with the community, which must be the foundation upon which community-based nursing education is built, was missing.

Interdisciplinary Efforts

The other element of the community-based definition that is difficult to articulate within the profession and difficult to achieve in the clinical arena is the notion of an interdisciplinary educational effort. It is evident to those who have worked with community projects that there is less domination by one profession in community settings than in more traditional hospital-based learning experiences. Nonetheless, by and large, nursing faculty continue to be parochial about who has the authority and the credentials to teach nursing students. (Ownership and control may be operative here as well!) Further, nursing faculty seem to be more reluctant to empower other health professionals to participate in the education of nursing students than other health professionals seem to be. Considerable work needs to be done to enable our students to work effectively with other health care providers in ways that transcend the boundaries of our traditional occupations.

PERCEIVED BARRIERS TO IMPLEMENTING COMMUNITY-BASED NURSING EDUCATION

Initiating a new project is always easier when one is aware of some of the barriers other have encountered. The barriers may be real or implied, based on fact or fears, easily overcome, or in need of a great deal of energy and negotiation to overcome. Understanding is the key to success.

Regulatory and Accreditation Issues

While defining the parameters of community-based nursing was an important component of the Visions II Project, an essential purpose was to identify, describe, and ultimately modify barriers to the implementation of such an educational approach. At the first consensus building meeting, significant barriers to community-based nursing education were proposed and discussed at length during all the sessions. This served as a tremendous opportunity to learn the regulations faculty perceived would prevent their efforts to move from the traditional hospital-based approaches to community-based education. The area in which there appeared to be considerable consensus was that the "Board," meaning the Boards of Registration in Nursing in Massachusetts and Rhode Island, and the "League," meaning the National League for Nursing Accrediting Commission, would not permit many of the approaches that the participants wanted to develop.

In response to these concerns, the second meeting included presentations from the NLN and the respective nursing boards (Massachusetts and Rhode Island). All emphasized their commitment to experimentation and their willingness to participate and support nursing educators and nursing programs who were engaged in innovation. On the basis of their statements, it was concluded that in Rhode Island and Massachusetts regulatory and accreditation barriers to community-based nursing education were minimal.

Pedagogical Concerns of Faculty

Most of the participants in the early meetings of the Visions II Project identified clear barriers based on the way they and most of their colleagues conceptualize clinical learning. There was a clear need for faculty to "rethink" how they approached nursing content and how they organized learning experiences. Yet, this task is difficult given the zeal with which old paradigms are embraced. Much of this stems from the way in which faculty have themselves been taught. Taglieri and Sherman (1997) cite the work of Bevis and Watson (1989) as acknowledging the way in which current faculty learned to be nurses. The process was "behavioral, content-laden, measurable, (within) a structured curriculum."

Consistent with this rather inflexible way of viewing clinical learning, it seemed as if the participants were invariably expressing grave concerns regarding the protection of their "license" and the legal implications of being responsible for students outside of their direct supervision. A number of their concerns reflect a lack of understanding on the part of some of the participants about their legal role in guiding student learning experiences.

It sometimes appears that faculty use concerns about legal issues as a deterrent against moving forward or making the kinds of changes that they are sometimes called upon to make. While it is true that the inability to provide direct supervision to all students in the clinical area is stressful to faculty, a comparison between those stresses in the acute care setting and those in the community arena appears to yield a high degree of similarity. Nonetheless, faculty clearly see the dispersion of students across a number of units or community agencies as limiting their ability to ensure the legal parameters of practice. It becomes apparent over time, in multiple conversations with participants and Task Force members, that faculty translate their own fears into legal consequences. They appear to do this with greater frequency when they are feeling uncertain and insecure.

Elements that faculty usually cite when expressing these concerns relate to their inability to directly observe all of the students' activities in the community setting. When making this comparison, it is common to forget just how infrequently students are directly observed in the acute care setting. In actuality, when a faculty member has 8-10 students in an acute care setting, the faculty is rarely, if ever, with more than one student at a time. What are the other 7-9 students doing? Based on our strong traditions in hospital-based services, as clinical instructors, we know of the checks and balances in that environment to assure that the patient is receiving the necessary attention. We do not possess similar understandings about routines and processes in the community settings. In addition, the notion of proximity which occurs when all of the students are engaged in their clinical learning at the same time, on the same unit, gives the faculty a sense of control and security (however, false!) that appears to be lost when they first move to the community. Due to the frequency in which I have heard this concern, it is clear that the comment reflects the degree to which the faculty is comfortable in the setting, not how comfortable the student is.

Furthermore, the participants noted that other tradeoffs formerly associated with community settings in the past no longer appear to be true, such as increase in acuity level in patient needs in the community. Often times the acuity level in the community is nearly as high as in the hospital. Faculty unfamiliar with the community are concerned about support in the event of untoward response of the patient. The faculty member who has spent his or her career in an environment in which help was as close as the call button is extremely unnerved by an environment in which help may be called on the phone, but delivery time is uncertain. Whether or not these issues are legal or related to a modification in preparation of faculty and/or their expectations of clinical learning remains to be seen.

Educational Preparation of Clinical Faculty

Another constant concern relates to the preparation of faculty for their role in the community and how this interfaced with existing requirements promulgated by the State Boards of Nursing and accrediting agencies. Specifically, each of these accrediting bodies requires a Master's degree in an area of clinical specialization in nursing for a faculty member to teach students preparing for licensure as a RN. Furthermore, it is specified that the faculty member must teach in his or her area of advanced preparation.

Clearly, these regulations and criteria were developed to ensure that students had access to faculty who possessed a level of knowledge that would foster student growth. Nonetheless, the question arises as to whether or not the Master's degree in an area of clinical specialization meets current needs for faculty positions. Is clinical specialty preparation congruent with an educational approach in undergraduate programs which emphasizes primary care, health promotion, and disease prevention in community-based settings? It may well be that a greater breadth of knowledge is necessary for an effective knowledge base for faculty in undergraduate education.

The role of the nurse in community-based settings appears to require a broader view more typical of the generalist than the specialist. The community-based practice of nursing is often delivered to the family unit. It is necessary for the nurse, and hence, the faculty to have a good understanding of developmental needs across the life cycle as well as insight into health measures and indices of disease in a much more comprehensive manner than a traditional clinical specialization provides.

Concomitantly, faculty are being called upon to further develop the science and craft of teaching. In an era marked by technological developments in pedagogical approaches and demanding greater efficiencies and effective outcomes from instruction, fewer and fewer nurse faculty are prepared to be educators.

The history of nursing education in the United States emanates from a strong orientation to the art of teaching, with the majority of the early leadership in nursing being prepared at advanced levels to be educators. Meanwhile, the period of time from the late 1960s through the 1980s witnessed an increased emphasis on specialization at the Master's level in nursing as the clinical practice arena became increasingly technological. The rise in acuity and the great strides made in lifesaving measures in the event of trauma or acute psychological assault led to significant expansion in the role of the nurse in the acute care setting, lending credence to the need for highly specialized work at the graduate level. As a result, graduate nursing education began to drop or severely limit programs of study to prepare nurses to function as educators. Currently, little time is available at the graduate level to teach about education, curriculum, student learning, or any of those elements of practice essential to the nurse interested in the art of teaching or wishing to develop an academic career. Since doctoral education in nursing is strongly rooted in research designs and methods, the development of leaders in education is a mounting void in the profession.

Faculty Performance Expectations

On the whole, the faculty participants in the Visions II Project possessed high expectations about their performance and seemed somewhat self critical. For example, the participants identified the need for faculty to have skills of creativity, flexibility, team membership, critical thinking and decision making, leadership, collaboration, and conflict resolution. This array of talent requirements appeared to reflect the faculty members' concerns about adjusting to a new environment and fulfilling the demands for modification in the education of nurses. It is evident that these faculty are being called upon to operationalize these skills in a new arena, one in which they lack a sense of confidence and security.

It has become evident that the profound and constant changes in the world of health care delivery, and the resultant modification in expectations for the graduate of nursing education programs, have occurred too quickly for the nursing education community to respond in a consistent and highly organized way. The commitment and talent of the faculty participants was apparent, yet their frustration with their own rate of learning and ability to adapt to the changes was equally obvious.

Faculty members are used to being experts, being confident about their approaches, and relish the satisfaction of joining their love of nursing practice with the joys of teaching. The degree and speed with which change has occurred has rocked the foundation of their practice, uprooted the site of their clinical expertise, and implies new expectations without pointing to a clear path for preparation. The passion with which the participants at the Vision II meetings expressed the barriers to moving forward was often based on inner-directed self-criticisms rather than objective assessments of the enormity and rapidity of change. Inherent in their comments were themes of powerlessness and perceived impotency in effecting the kinds of changes that they believe need to occur and considerable personal hesitation to move forward.

Security in the Traditions of Nursing Education

Coupling faculty's concern and lack of confidence with nursing education's historic prescriptive nature allows the dimensions of the problems for our new world of education to become clearer. Traditionally, nursing education has been heavily vested in the presentation of facts that are! Marginal time has been allocated to opportunities for discussion of dilemmas or analysis of complex clinical incidents that may be. Nurse educators, collectively, have for too long been vested in the direct transmission of a body of content to be recalled and repeated by students and in using the clinical setting to enable the student to demonstrate what he/she has learned. (During all of my professional career I have been mystified about where students actually learn, since evidence of "not knowing" in the clinical setting is traditionally associated with being "unprepared.") All of these elements have historically given clear direction and focus to the educational mission, for nursing faculty as much as for nursing students.

The present environment calls for a different approach and skill set for faculty, yet training for uncertainty has not been part of the traditions of nursing education. Hence, it is not surprising that the faculty allude so frequently to the authority structures as deterrents in their exploration of alternative educational approaches. When any individual or group embarks on new ventures, they need some rules or guidelines to set the stage. When these are lacking, when the terror of the times is filled with uncertainty, old rules become even more important.

Fortunately, however, it appears as if participation in the discussions of the Visions II Project had a powerful effect on these faculty members, an outcome that provides direction for future planning. First, the Visions II meetings provided faculty with the opportunity to learn and see how pervasive the challenge of community-based education is. Second, and of equal importance, they learned that they were not alone in their feelings of inadequacy and together explored ways to work with others and overcome those barriers. Over the course of the five meetings, there was a palpable change in the level of confidence, with the gradual appearance of enthusiasm and a "can do" attitude.

As educators and health professionals, we all know that there is an optimal level of stress at which student learning is enhanced. When the stress continues to develop it can pass a point at which learning becomes impaired. This knowledge also applies to faculty learning. At the outset, it was most evident that the level of faculty insecurity with the changing environment was significant and functioning as a deterrent to their growth and development related to community-based nursing education. As faculty issues, concerns, and implications were discussed, they came to realize that they knew a great deal more about community-based education than they were aware of or credited themselves for, and they started to relax.

At the final bi-state meeting of the project it was evident that understanding and sensitivity to the process of community-based nursing education had increased remarkably from the first meeting. Faculty learning had been additive; the more experience individuals had with community-based teaching and learning, the more they liked about it, and the more its underpinnings became clear to them. Hence, learning about community-based nursing education is a process.

Administrative Issues

There was considerable overlap between the things that were of concern to faculty and the administrative and professional implications. In some items the difference between the two related to the perspective. This was particularly evident with regard to legal issues. For the most part, however, the barriers identified here are issues of the faculty that have significant administrative implications. For example, when faculty lament their need for professional development to function well in the community setting, the administration of the nursing program must respond with the resources to assist the faculty to achieve what they need to move forward.

Many of the concerns voiced by the participants indicated considerable insecurity over the support and recognition they could count on receiving from their educational administrators. The concern about this aspect of support was widespread, was not associated with any particular level or type of nursing education, and did not appear to be substantially relieved at the end of the project. There was good attendance from the educational administrators, but determination was not of the degree to which the concerns of the faculty were an accurate reflection of the perception of the administrators or the misguided perception of the faculty.

Faculty express fear of a lack of administrative support whereas administrators often lament the resistance of faculty to change. It is essential to the advancement of the discipline of nursing that the ineffective dynamics of mutual blaming be eliminated and replaced with a clear articulation of the relative demands of the respective roles in faculty and academic administration.

Assurance of Quality Learning Experiences

There are a number of items that fell into this category, most reflecting the insecurity of the faculty in the new domain of community. For example, the faculty expressed concern about client confidentiality. It appeared as if the participants saw the parameters of patient/client confidentiality as greater than, or different from, the parameters in the institutional setting. These concerns seemed to be greatest in the small communities where there was a higher probability of patient/client lives intersecting with the professionals' lives on many levels. Concern about the ability of beginning students to behave responsibly as they learn the nuances of the professional role may have serious implications for the development of community experiences.

The inability to predict viability of care settings is another faculty concern which may have administrative implications. Clinical learning activities often fall through in these times of change in patient care arena. In community-based services, a number of programs are funded on a short-term basis and provide short-term commitments to clients. As a result, there is a dimension of fluidity about learning experiences in the community that is less predictable than traditional in-patient experiences. The implications for students learning with these unpredictable flows in patient care clearly challenges the faculty. The participants perceived that ultimately this burden should land back on the shoulders of the administrator.

Currently, there is also increasing inconsistency in patient census in the acute care sector and mounting concerns about assuring quality learning experiences in any health care arena. The *Essential Clinical Resources for Nursing's Academic Mission* (AACN, 1999) spells out these issues clearly and identifies potential sources of change.

Attention to the way in which the presence of students effects costs of services is being closely examined in all clinical sectors and was frequently mentioned by the participants in the Visions II Project. For example, many of the large medical centers formerly employed a person full-time to interface between the nursing administration of the hospital and the educational institutions. More commonly now, these tasks are simply absorbed by a member of human resources, not necessarily a nurse. In community-based settings where parameters for students experiences may be a new initiative, processes of incorporating the student may not be in place, or their development is compromised by constraints of time, given the mandate to fill all patient care sessions with direct patient care services. Hence, the organization and planning for clinical learning experiences has become more burdensome for faculty in all settings. It is critical that administrators and faculty solve problems in proactive, collaborative ways to address these pressing concerns.

Expectations of Preparation: Educational Arena vs. Practice Arena

The nature and pace of changes in the clinical arena have created a highly volatile environment for all, including the administrators of nursing education programs. Nursing education and nursing service have long been differentiated on the basis of their mission with nursing education future-oriented and nursing practice focused on the present. Historically, nursing service has informed nursing education about the requirements needed by our graduates to function as professional nurses. It has been the impression of many educators that the demand for a finished product in the entry level of the profession was unrealistic. At the present time, however, there is a perception that nursing service has even increased its demands and expectations for the new graduate. Coupling pressures to expand the domain of practice sites and related content that nurses are dealing with in the community, nursing service administrators continue to also add topics that new graduates must have. Among these are competence in knowledge about the reimbursement system and implications for nursing care services, policies of the diverse managed care plans including Medicare and Medicaid, and managing patient care needs within these constraints.

PARTNERSHIPS WITH HOSPITAL NURSING SERVICES

As faculty began to give attention to the need to explore and develop new relationships with clinical sites, they specifically advocated the establishment of partnerships with communities. What was startling was the failure of any of the work groups to note that nursing education has rarely entered into a genuine partnership with the nursing services of agencies. The more common belief in the hospital arena is that nursing service ought to accommodate the needs of the educational programs—an entitlement to access. When the faculty start to develop new relationships and ways of interacting in spheres of practice within which they are less comfortable, such as the community, they are more conscious of the contribution of the community agencies and exhibit less of a sense of entitlement.

Another awareness was that the community must have some direct input into the nature of the learning experiences of students and the kind of curriculum being offered. While nurse educators and nursing service personnel have long met to discuss the needed attributes of the graduates, the extent to which nursing service has directly influenced the development of curriculum is unclear.

The nursing literature has long lamented the schism between education and service. Within the discussions of the Visions II Project, the participants from both nursing service and nursing education appeared to gain sensitivity to each other's framework and the pressures each work under. This awareness needs to be strengthened to broaden the sphere of influence of nursing and focus on combining our energies for the improvement of nursing.

Curriculum and Clinical Practice Issues

Within the context of the Visions II Project there was limited discussion of curriculum content. Many lamented the problems associated with finding viable learning experiences for students in the area of obstetrics. This exemplifies the conflict between following the medical model and transferring the quest for learning experiences from one arena to another rather than developing the content for a curriculum and clinical experiences based on the learning needs of students. The questions to be asked is, "Are future nurses best served by learning more about women during the prenatal and postpartum period, which nurses in a variety of positions encounter, or by focusing on the in-hospital care which is a specialty area in which very few nurses provide care?

The majority of the discussion related to curriculum focused on ways in which content could be organized and presented in different ways. Primarily, the object of attention was the organization of student learning experiences. Faculty expressed ambivalence about implementing more traditional hospital-based experiences while they simultaneously tried to learn about communities. They recognized that the nature of interactions in the clinical area would need to change. Although they could clearly espouse a commitment to developing new kinds of relationships with community-based clinical agencies, the inexperienced in community-based partnerships could not readily identify what they would be like.

Clinical Learning Sites

The centrality of concern about the quality of clinical learning experiences was both a product of faculty expertise, as in barriers related to faculty, and in the availability of resources within the community. Faculty were concerned about the amount of time it would take to locate clinical sites in the community, coupled with the substantial planning that occurs once a partnership is established.

Participants verbalized considerable difficulty in the accurate assessment of the value of particular types of learning experiences. In acknowledging the increasing difficulties of in-patient clinical placements, there appeared to be a degree of comfort in knowing that a majority of the experiences in the hospital interface in some direct manner with the content of a given course. There was not this level of comfort in community placements. This point may exemplify ambivalence some faculty feel about the value of health promotion learning activities. In addition they appear to have considerable trouble deciding if a community agency has the ingredients that will create a positive learning experience and an environment in which student knowledge will flourish.

In addition, faculty reported considerable down time in community settings. (Down time refers to those times over the course of a clinical period in which the students does not have clearly identifiable tasks in which to engage.) There is, however, a parallel in hospital clinical experiences waiting for one thing or another to happen. Perhaps it was waiting for the x-rays to return, or the MD to show up, or the operating room schedule to be posted, or the visitor to leave. The point is that there are an array of activities that hold up student activities in the hospital. The ones in the community are just new. As faculty experience in community-based education grew the amount of down time of students decreased and their ability to relate the experiences to student's ultimate career goals increased.

Student safety in community-based settings, and the belief of faculty that they are responsible for ensuring the physical safety of students was another frequent curriculum theme. Faculty also had concerns about their own safety. While there is no pat answer for these concerns in this notoriously unsafe age, there does seem to be a correlation between safety concerns and degree of experience, awareness, and comfort of the community. Safety concerns are expressed more often by faculty who had not yet ventured into the communities. Participants who did have experience in the community did not see danger as a deterrent and believed that the overwhelming majority of the communities are basically safe when appropriate measures are taken. Perhaps the faculty who had gone into the community were able to discern the difference between an underserved, low income area and an unsafe area.

Finally, faculty verbalized a sense of loss of control over the quality or nature of the student learning experiences in community settings. This concern is articulated with respect to the faculty's ability to influence when or how health care is delivered in community-based settings. While this observation may be true, one is struck by the inference that nursing faculty somehow control learning experiences in other settings. It is perhaps an accompaniment of new endeavors that the old ways appear to be somehow safer, or more in concert with long-held values. Or, if the truth be told, the values have been shaped by the environment. The reality, however, is that nursing faculty have always articulated frustration at not being able to control events within clinical settings, hospitals, nursing homes, etc.

It may be that faculty felt a semblance of control in more traditional settings because they were experienced and sufficiently confident with the mechanics of the organizations. In reality staff nurses often indicate which patients are available to students or who would be willing to have a student provide their care. Regardless of the personal beliefs of the faculty in that clinical site, it would be rare to disagree with the recommendations from the staff. Hence, lack of control of clinical learning experiences is not new.

As faculty become more knowledgeable about a community with its range of services and learning opportunities, their comfort level is likely to increase. The theme related to perceived power abated over the course of the project, with the participants expressing growing optimism about working with other groups and feeling capable of influencing outcomes in the revised healthcare system.

Restraints on Community/Providers

IMPOSITION ON TIME OF PRACTICING NURSES

Nursing service participants in the project reported on a diversity of issues that effect their ability to collaborate in ways comparable to the past, and lamented mounting pressure on them to assess the financial impact of involvement in nursing education programs. Specifically they noted that reimbursement is clearly tied to disease management, not health promotion activities. The demands of the present reimbursement system negatively effect all efforts to engage in working with student groups.

The requirements related to contracts, health clearances, felony checks and the plethora of details that plague educational programs have an impact on the agencies in which the students have clinical experiences. Just as these requirements impinge on educators, they create work place demands on providers.

FAILURE TO DIFFERENTIATE COMPETENCIES

Within the community arena there are no models of practice that accommodate differing levels of education. Graduates of all nursing programs leading to licensure as an RN are competing for employment in the same job pool, as human resource managers do not always understand the differing ways the graduates have been educated. Associate degree program graduates are entering the job market in community-based jobs, and employers are expecting these graduates to possess a level of knowledge that even the baccalaureate programs cannot assure. Community-based roles for licensed practical nurses (LPNs) have long existed, and many new opportunities are developing along these lines without reference to their educational experiences. Employers cite the failure of nursing education to identify a comprehensive difference between the graduates with respect to competencies, while nurse educators cite the lack of realism in the expectations for all new graduates.

LACK OF CONSISTENCY IN CLIENT CARE

Employers of nurses cite lack of consistency in client care in the community as a critical problem which is worsened when students are added to the mix. Providers identify the constant introduction of new individuals to clients as difficult for clients and staff and time consuming for the agency. According to the participants from the service sector, nursing education must identify some ways in which continuity of students' experiences can be developed to provide smoother working relationships with agencies and client groups.

Evaluation of Student Clinical Performance

Concern for quality student learning experiences while ensuring quality patient care service has been the hallmark of nursing education since its inception and was well-articulated within this project. Faculty on the traditional community courses have considerable experience in evaluating students' learning. Faculty new to the community-based concepts, however, expressed specific concerns when working in the community sector. These are summarized below.

Significant discussion was raised about quality control issues that stem from the nature of the learning experience. The process that needs to be developed must include the establishment of attainable and measurable outcome behaviors that relate to the adequacy of experiences in terms of number, variety, and placement. Mechanisms also need to be discovered to assist us in studying with more precision the nature of clinical learning. Only when the phenomenon is clearly understood will we be able to make sound decisions about the need for and role of faculty in the clinical area. Is it supervision or is it mentoring? Can it be accomplished through the work of a preceptor, with faculty support, or are strong clinical nurses the best clinical teachers? We do not have the answers to these questions.

Couples with these concerns are the barriers faculty face in attempting to assess student learning. While patient safety is a serious consideration, faculty are also concerned about how they can validate what students have learned and how they can rate that learning according to some measurable criteria. This has long been an issue and is not new with community-based nursing education. The shift in the clinical environment has just brought the discussion to the forefront again.

The primary dilemma about evaluating the impact of the student experience on learning is the lack of consensus we have in nursing education about what constitutes a strong learning experience. Faculty often romanticize traditional learning experiences as they see that world being dismantled. Comparable to the losses articulated by staff, faculty allude to the good old days when patient care services appeared to be more focused on services needed rather than the cost of the care. There is a tendency to forget the elements in that world that did not work.

Faculty lament that in the community they are not able to fully monitor the work of the students. A few of us remember the days of the large wards with 20 or more patients in a room, when simultaneous observation of all students and patients was possible. Those days have been absent for some time. For many years, faculty have had to depend on the assistance of staff to guide students and to interpret outcomes of care.

The remedy to these barriers rests in the very first one identified which relates to faculty's ability to re-think nursing education. Most nursing faculty continue to conceptualize curriculum and student learning along a linear dimension. Nursing education has traditionally been organized with content sequentially developed and concepts presented from simple to complex. There is increasing evidence based on the explosion of technology and the resultant application within education that people do not necessarily learn in a linear fashion. The use of computers in education has shown that students can "plug in and plug out" at different places with different types of learning occurring along the way. The process of nursing education should respond to the research and develop more along these lines.

Students' Beliefs About Nursing

Students enter our programs with a certain perception of nursing practice. Clearly, the dramatized and public view of the nurse continues to be problematic for the profession. With the general public poorly informed, based on widespread misinterpretation of the role of the nurse, the public relations issues within nursing are significant. For the man or woman seeking a career in nursing, the source of information is rooted in the past or in commonly held notions about nursing practice. Most of these are founded on a view of a nurse in a hospital, hence, locating nursing education experiences in a community conflicts with the students preconceived notions and is sometimes poorly received.

In addition, the allure of the high-tech world of acute care has not been matched with a highly visible role model in the community sector. Examples of successful nurses in arenas outside the hospital parameters need to be discovered and fostered. Reading *Life Support* (Gordon, 1997) may start this process of enlightenment.

In a comparable vein, the early desire of nursing students to develop skills in the techniques of practice remains prevalent. Ways must be discerned to allow attention to the performance of the technical skills of nursing in the community setting as it meets some of their needs for tangible evidence of progress in learning about nursing.

MOVING TOWARD THE FUTURE

The primary contribution of the Visions II Project to the nursing community in the two-state area appears to have been the provision of a forum to explore the issues and concerns surrounding community-based nursing education. It provided that forum in a way that maximized the ability of nurse educators, students, and nursing service personnel to share ideas and collaborate without interference. The participants met the challenge with creativity, enthusiasm, and a genuine commitment to translate ideas into specific learning opportunities for students.

Twenty-two projects were initiated and developed within different schools in the bi-state area. Among the strengths of the projects are:

- interdisciplinary teamwork
- collaboration with service providers
- strong relationships between schools and regulatory bodies
- recognition that student experiences are no longer generic or homogeneous

These projects supplied the same closure to the full circle of learning that this book exemplifies. By sharing the diverse programs that have been successfully implemented based on the principles of community-based nursing education, a sense of communion is fostered that is so essential to the development of the profession.

The development of genuine and comprehensive partnerships between health care providers in all settings and health professions education is the key to successful preparation of the next generation of health professionals. There is no question that we have considerable work to do in refining and building our community partnerships to enhance student learning. We can accomplish that as we nurture our collective creative talent. Regardless of the setbacks, nursing faculty members are "can do" people who overcome the difficulties and grow in the challenge. The generous sharing of programs within this book will inspire you to new ventures and new rewards.

REFERENCES

American Nurses Association (ANA). (1986). *Standards of Community Health Nursing Practice*. (ANA Pub. No. CH-2) Washington, DC: Author.

American Nurses Association (ANA). (1990). *Nursing's Agenda for Health Care Reform*. Washington, DC: Author.

American Association of Colleges of Nursing (AACN). (1997). *A Vision of Baccalaureate and Graduate Nursing Education: the Next Decade*. Washington, DC: Author.

American Association of Colleges of Nursing (AACN). (1998). *The Essentials of Baccalaureate Education for Professional Nursing Practice*. Washington, DC: Author.

American Association of Colleges of Nursing (AACN). (1999). *Essential Clinical Resources for Nursing's Academic Mission*. Washington, DC: Author.

American Public Health Association (APHA). (1981). *The definition and role of public health nursing practice in the delivery of health care: A statement of the public health nursing section*. Washington, DC: Author.

National League of Nursing. (1993). *A vision for nursing education*. New York: Author.

National League of Nursing. (1997). *Visions II community-based nursing education project. Final Report*. New York: Author.

Pew Health Professions Commission. (1991). *Healthy American: Practitioners for 2005: An agenda for action for health professions schools*. Durham, NC: Author.

Tagliareni, M. E. & Markx, B. B. (1997). *Teaching in the Community: Preparing Nurses for the 21st Century*. New York: NLN.

3

In The Shadow Of A Mouse All Is Not A Magic Kingdom: The Experience at the University of Central Florida

Ermalynn Kiehl

When most people think of Orlando, Florida, they think about Walt Disney World and the entertainment and recreation activities available. Prior to the arrival of the Walt Disney Company in the 1960s, agriculture was the primary source of employment with plentiful crops of citrus, fern, and vegetables. The construction of the Disney World complex provided many more jobs in the area, and many families moved to Orlando from around the country. In addition to Disney, Universal Studios and Sea World occupy land that once grew oranges, and employees' houses have risen where the carrots and cabbage grew. The influx of residents continues as many other companies find the climate, the pool of cheap labor, and the established tourist base a desirable asset.

Central Florida is among the nation's top 10 fastest growing metropolitan areas, according to the U.S. Census Bureau. The growth rate of Central Florida was 7.8% between 1990–1994, approximately 2.5 times the rate for the U.S. as a whole. The Central Florida counties include Orange, Seminole, and Brevard.

Orange County is the heart of Central Florida and the location of the main campus of the University of Central Florida. Orange County has over 675,000 residents. As in most metropolitan areas, Orange County has a diverse population. Orange County public schools list over 100 languages spoken by children entering the school system.

Seminole County is located in North Central Florida. It has a population of over 287,529. Seminole County is considered the "bedroom" community of Orlando with large pockets of affluent residential and commercial areas. Yet, it also is home to some of the lowest per-capita income families in Florida.

Brevard County is located in East Central Florida. It is 70 miles long and approximately 25 miles wide and is bordered by the Atlantic Ocean and the St. Johns River. The population is 398,978. This county is mainly rural with some suburbs. There are no large municipalities.

Health care for these three counties is provided by four major hospital systems. Although all of these systems provide some care to the medically underserved of the county, most do so on the grounds of the acute care facility. Home health services are primarily provided by these same systems.

In addition, each area has a County Health Department which provides services to individuals who have completed the Medicaid eligibility process. Services are provided to pregnant women and preschool children. Adult services are limited to international immunizations and management of tuberculosis and sexually transmitted diseases including HIV/AIDS.

Orlando is typical of other cities in the Sunbelt as its population continues to expand at the rapid rate of 14% per year. There is a large influx of immigrants from ethnically and culturally diverse minority groups. In the Orlando area, minorities comprise approximately 40.3%, in contrast to 27.6% of the population nationally. Major ethnic groups originate from South and Central America, Haiti, the Caribbean islands, and Asia. In addition, Central Florida has experienced an influx of elderly retirees from across the country as well as young families in search of opportunities within the exploding technological, entertainment, and service industries. The media presents a uniform and radiant picture of Central Florida, so it is hard to imagine the number of culturally and linguistically diverse neighborhoods and many medically undeserved families that exist in Central Florida. Behind the advertised façade lies the fact that Orlando is a typical metropolitan area facing rapid expansion, a diverse immigrant and ethnic population, and major health care disparities.

Access to health care is increasingly difficult for residents in the lower socioeconomic areas of the city of Orlando and other areas of Central Florida. Barriers including transportation and work schedules that make access to health care impossible for an increasing number of people.

One of Our Neighborhoods

One underserved neighborhood exists literally in the shadow of International Drive, an ornate tourist area with endless hotels, restaurants, and activities next to Disney World. Two blocks from this drive is Tangelo Park with approximately 2,600 residents. The neighborhood is comprised of cement block homes that once housed workers from a defense plant. With urban expansion encroaching on the neighborhood and financial success, the upwardly mobile population moved to larger suburban homes, leaving this community to become home to low-income renters and impoverished families.

Within this neighborhood is one church, a YMCA, and an elementary school. Greater than 90% of the students receive free or reduced fee lunches. The community is devoid of any major health care services with the exception of emergency services provided at the fire station. The nearest health care provider is eight miles away.

At the entrance to Tangelo Park is a convenience store that carries delicatessen-type items, sodas, and beer. The convenience store also sells used cars and, at night, hosts drug activity. The other commercial establishment is a Texaco station that sells similar items. While fast food is readily available, the availability of fresh fruits, vegetables, meat, or dairy products is at least a 15-minute car ride or a two-hour, one-way bus trip away. Access to public transportation is very restricted and involves a trip to a central station and transfer to another bus to reach a particular destination.

Tangelo Park is 92% African-American, many of who are in poor health. The incidence of diabetes (9.9%) is more than three times the national (2.8%) average. The rate of death from AIDS is 7.4% more than double that of the national average (3.2%).

Establishing A Clinical Home

With space available in the school, a partnership was established between the Orange County Public School System and the University of Central Florida (UCF) to begin to provide the basic health care services of health promotion and preventative screening for this neighborhood. The project is called the Tangelo Park—University of Central Florida Community Nursing Center (CNC).

After conducting an initial community assessment, the junior nursing students assigned to this neighborhood surveyed the school children. The survey revealed that these young children had major concerns about such things as guns, fire, and drug activity. To begin to address these concerns the nursing students developed a learning tool for the children. In the book, a puppy with big eyes and a Band-Aid on his bottom winds his way from page to page facing the dangers the children had identified and making choices that keep the puppy safe. The children responded well to the book and talked about applying the decisions the puppy made to their own situations.

Having met with initial success and starting to feel a relationship developing with the residents, the nursing students prioritized the other needs they had identified during the community assessment. They developed programs with residents of all ages and provided health care by:

- initiating a "Jump-Start Awareness Project" to encourage language development, spatial and motion awareness, and gross and fine motor development
- teaching hygiene and nutrition principles to kindergarten and first graders as a part of a reading project
- using principles of hygiene and nutrition while teaching word and number recognition
- developing and presenting a safety program for children who practice self-care
- providing health education about chronic illness management, monitoring health changes, and proper use of common medications including side effects, risks, and danger signs for senior citizens
- conducting a Health Fair that included individual teaching projects that demonstrated nutrition management, cancer detection and screening activities, exercise, and stress management
- developing a culturally sensitive diabetes brochure that was circulated to the clients in the local community church
- monitoring 12–20 senior citizens weekly for chronic conditions

Through these activities, the nursing students encouraged language development and self-confidence in the children and adults while sharing useful information to help in their daily lives.

In addition to the undergraduate generic students, graduate students and undergraduate RN-BSN students also shared their skills. Students in the Family Nurse Practitioner Program participated in the school readiness project and Family Health Fair in conjunction with Tangelo Baptist Church family day. The undergraduate RN-BSN students participated in the Health Fair and community assessment.

NEIGHBORHOOD-BASED CLINICAL EDUCATION

A neighborhood-based community education program brings together the members of academia, faculty, and students with the people of the neighborhood, both providers and residents. They collaborate in the assessment of the neighborhood and then develop an implementation strategy to address health care issues.

The Academic Partners

The University of Central Florida (UCF) is one of the 10 universities in the Florida State University System. Founded in 1963 as Florida Technological University, the name was changed in 1978 to the University of Central Florida. There are more than 28,000 enrolled in its five colleges. The university is located on 1445 acres, 13 miles northeast of downtown Orlando.

The School of Nursing (SON) initially accredited in the fall of 1981 is part of the College of Health and Public Affairs, a relatively new college which brings together a variety of programs in the health and public affairs fields. In addition to the main campus, the SON has satellite campuses in Daytona Beach, Cocoa, Downtown Orlando, and the Orlando Regional Healthcare System. Classes are also held at the Lake Sumter Community College in Leesburg, Florida for RN-BSN bridge students.

THE NURSING STUDENTS

The diversity of the Orlando metropolitan area is reflected in the student body. The SON serves many different groups of students—working commuter students, non-traditional students, women with families returning to school, first generation college students, second degree students, and ethnic and cultural sub-populations with special needs as well as traditional and residential students.

Approximately 400 applications are received at the SON for 70 student placements each year. Due to this competition, applicants are placed in rank order-based 60% on their GPA and 40% on their nursing program prerequisite grades.

Students at the University of Central Florida represent many educational pathways. Students might be recent high school graduates for which this is their first time in college or individuals who have completed prior course work which may have resulted in receipt of a diploma in nursing or an Associate's degree in Science or in Arts, a Baccalaureate, or graduate degrees.

VISION OF THE FACULTY

The faculty of the School of Nursing believes that a community-based approach to nursing care delivery is essential for educating the nurse of the future and that community-based primary care concepts must be taught and practiced by immersing students within various local neighborhoods. Immersion allows the students and the University community with the opportunity to form collaborative partnerships.

GOALS OF THE UNDERGRADUATE PROGRAM

1. To prepare nurses who can effect positive outcomes in health and health care
2. To educate nurses whose contributions:
   • increase knowledge among clients and client systems about the nature of health problems, normal growth and development, and avenues for intervention
   • enhance the capacity for problem-solving and decision-making among consumers and health care providers
   • intervene in the trajectory of illness and lived experiences with health problems among clients and client systems by maximizing human potential, growth, and healing
   • improve the responsiveness, accessibility, efficiency, and effectiveness of the health care system
   • provide access to quality preventative health, community-based care, and quality nursing services across the continuum of care for clients and families
3. To provide students the opportunity to practice nursing within a community-based approach to the delivery and evaluation of care

Bringing about Change

Until 1995, the nursing program model at the UCF School of Nursing (SON) was a traditional model in which the student's education was focused primarily towards acute care nursing. Although there was a community health course in the fall of the student's senior year and various community experiences throughout several other courses such as the childbearing and childrearing family and psychiatric nursing, the program design essentially socialized the students for acute care nursing.

When faculty began to consider a curriculum revision, guest speakers on curriculum change and community-based curricula were invited to present seminars. Most faculty members agreed that change needed to occur but no one knew exactly how to bring about a change, or to what degree, or in what way? [A complete timeline of faculty activities appears in Table 3-1.]

TABLE 3-1 Time Line for New Curriculum Implementation

7/96	Faculty member attended Northeastern University Summer Institute: Nursing in the Neighborhoods
8/96	Faculty retreat was conducted to discuss the Northeastern nursing education program and get agreement of UCFSON direction
8/96	Faculty member identified to direct curriculum redesign and implementation
9–11/96	Full faculty meetings to outline curriculum redesign. Group work for vision, mission, goals, conceptual framework, and undergraduate curriculum overview
1–3/97	Faculty divides in teams and works on individual semesters
3/97	Faculty agrees with detailed proposed curriculum revision
4/97	Met with the UCFSON Community Advisory to detail proposed curriculum redesign
4/97	Met with newly accepted Junior students to discuss the new curriculum
5–6/97	Investigated possible partnerships and sites
6/97	Presented curriculum and received approval from BON
6/97	Presented redesigned curriculum to educators and administrators from local acute care institutions*
6/97	Presented redesigned curriculum to Florida Organization of Nurse Executives
7/97	Sent letters to newly accepted Junior students re: selecting neighborhood sites
8/97	Began new curriculum

* Very important since they hired students as Nurse Techs after a certain point in the old curriculum. Since this "point" would no longer exist, the institutions would need to revise their policies and potentially their orientation regarding nursing student employees.

In the fall of 1997, the student body consisted of 67 junior and 75 senior students in the basic program, 258 RN-BSN students, and 55 graduate students. Graduates of the baccalaureate nursing program who are not already registered nurses are eligible to sit for licensure examination as Registered Nurses. Generic pass rate on the NCLEX is 97% to 100%.

About that time, a brochure arrived announcing a Summer Institute for "Nursing in the Neighborhoods" at Northeastern University in Boston. Perhaps some ideas could be derived from this workshop. One faculty member was selected to attend the Summer Institute. During the visit to Boston, the UCF faculty became convinced that the principles of this model would work for the University of Central Florida School of Nursing. The information gained during participation in the Summer Institute ultimately provided the framework for the curriculum change.

Upon her return, an all faculty retreat was held to share the concepts learned at the Summer Institute. The retreat began by sharing the metaphor of "The Ocean" (Shea, 1995). Essentially, the metaphor compares the ocean to primary health care. Students come to this challenging experience with a variety of expectations and experiences with which to handle the encounter.

For most the ocean is vast, mysterious, and frightening. The pond swimmers are used to well-contained banks, consistent waterline, and a predictable depth. They are surprised to learn that the ocean has a varied shoreline, constantly changing tides, and BIG waves. But, they like the sandy bottom, and the buoyancy of the salt water. They like to ride the waves, once they are not afraid. They learned to take advantage of the power of the ocean, and they became strong swimmers.

The pool swimmers are surprised to find that the ocean shoreline stretched to the farthest horizon, the salt air smelled much better than chlorine, and there were no time-consuming pool cleaning chores! But they were bothered by their inability to control the temperature of the water. The water wasn't crystal clear so they couldn't see the bottom, and they didn't like to deal with the salt and sticky sand.

The non-swimmers had no experience with swimming except what they had seen on television. They were captivated by the natural beauty of the ocean—the sights, the sounds, the smells, and the breeze. They found it so refreshing. It seemed to clean itself by washing things out to sea, returning treasures. But they didn't dive right in like the pool swimmers did, but rather they waded in slowly. They learned to carefully step among the shells and, in time, they respected the power of the ocean and enjoyed its bounty.

Students and faculty will have professional preferences. Some will like the ocean (community-based primary care). Others will prefer the swimming pool (hospital-based tertiary care). Students need ample, guided experiences in both to understand the complexities of health care. The community, just as the Ocean, is a powerful natural entity. It commands strong feelings, requires special skills, and offers boundless opportunities for education, research, and service (Shea, 1995).

Several points considered by the faculty during the retreat were:
- the current health care system with very short patient stays in acute care facilities
- the morale of the acute care nurses due to downsizing
- the increasing competition for clinical placements
- the lack of clinical placements restricting the number of students UCF could admit

The faculty agreed that, as health care shifted from hospital care to more primary care and preventative services, the health care system requires registered nurses who are prepared to practice in multiple settings and who possess clinical decision-making, case management skills and skills in health promotion and preventative and long-term care. The faculty agreed in principle with the recommendations of the Pew Health Professions Commission (1995), the American Association of Colleges of Nursing (1996), the Association of Nurse Executive (1996), and the National League for Nursing (1998). Each organization supported the idea that preparation of entry-level professional nurses required greater orientation to community-based primary care and emphasis on health promotion, maintenance, and cost-effective, coordinated care.

The retreat ended with challenging quotes from Dr. Carl Hammerschlag (Personal communication, 1995), including:

- Success is a leap of faith.
- If you have to know what you'll do before you do it, then you'll only do what you've already done.
- If you have to know where it is that you're going before you go, then you'll only get where you've already been.
- The only things we know are those we've already done; everything else is a guess.

Although specifics about just how to design the program remained open at the close of this first retreat, the faculty member who had attended the Summer Institute was identified as the Curriculum Coordinator, responsible for facilitating the curriculum revision and implementation.

The faculty knew that designing a new curriculum with a community orientation was essential. To ensure that they built the new curriculum on a cohesive foundation, the faculty developed a new vision, mission, goals, conceptual framework, and then an overview of an undergraduate curriculum.

Their actions were based on the belief that a community-based approach to nursing care delivery is essential for educating the nurse of the future. Community-based primary care concepts must be taught and practiced with individuals, families, and groups. Immersing students within various local neighborhoods provides the students and the UCF community the opportunity to form collaborative partnerships. The purpose is to not only educate students but to also effect positive health outcomes of neighborhood residents. The major concepts to include are systems, health, nursing, and nursing's clients. The sub-concepts are culture, ethics, and values. Learning threads are epidemiology, diagnostic reasoning, communication, and collaboration.

The Community-based Curriculum

Course work and clinical experiences flow from healthy to acutely ill. During the *first semester of Year I*, students are introduced to the community as the framework for understanding the functioning of families and the epidemiological basis of health and health events. Content areas included in this semester are lifespan approaches to health promotion and epidemiological approaches to community health assessment within the national context of Healthy People 2000 Goals. The focus of clinical content includes diagnostic reasoning, therapeutic communication, application of assessment strategies, multicultural sensitivity, community assessment, and nursing care of families experiencing normal developmental events and minor, self-limiting health concerns. The content and clinical experiences build initial knowledge and skills needed to work as a professional nurse within a community-based framework for nursing practice.

The *second semester of Year I* focuses on promoting physical and mental health. Content and clinical experiences are related to core knowledge and skills needed by nurses for practice in all settings and include pharmacology and pathophysiology in addition to physical and mental health and clinical practice. Building on foundational knowledge of health promotion, the student integrates a holistic model of nursing practice for individuals and families experiencing health risks, chronic health problems, or short-term illness, with simultaneous concern for mental and physical health needs emphasized. A biopsychosocial approach is developed with increasing consideration for social, ethical, economic, and legal aspects of health and nursing services. In the summer session, the focus is on "The Science of Nursing Practice." In this semester, the student takes the Nursing Research course and an elective. These non-clinical nursing courses build an understanding of the scientific and expert basis of nursing as a discipline.

The focus of the *first semester of Year II*, is on Nursing Care in Acute and Life Threatening Illness across the life span, when the family is no longer able to care for the individual at home and acute care is needed. The content of didactic and clinical courses covers the nursing care of individuals and families undergoing acute and life threatening physical or mental illness. The function of the nurse in the context of health care systems is addressed in "Leadership and Management" where the student explores the nursing practice environment, including support for direct service, delegated practice models, interdisciplinary and collaborative approaches to health care, and management and evaluation for health services delivery.

The focus of the *final semester during Year II* is nurse as change agent and case manager for health care in the community. Working within a community-based practice model to effect changes in the health status, health risk, and self-care capacity of target populations is practiced in a variety of settings. Intervening at the community level to effect health outcomes is supported by the "Health Care Issues, Policy, and Economics," "Role Transition," and "Community as the Continuum of Care" courses. The "Practicum" course provides an opportunity for the student to integrate experiences in the program, evolve role entry-level proficiency, and focus career goals. [See Table 3-2 for details].

THE STUDENTS

All students admitted to the nursing program are expected to complete clinical rotations within their "assigned" neighborhood. Students accepted into the program are sent a letter with a short general description of each center. They are given the opportunity to select their first, second, and third choices. Although most students get their first choice (60%), some difficulty occurs when more students request the Brevard Center than can be accommodated. As a result, some students have to drive approximately 30 miles into Orange County for their clinical experiences. In spite of this hardship for a certain group of students, they accept it optimistically.

Community Partners in Education

The School of Nursing (SON) faculty agreed that a total of seven Community Nursing Centers (CNCs) would be needed to accommodate the 70 nursing students admitted each year. Although the Florida Board of Nursing allows 12 students to be assigned to one faculty for clinical experiences, the SON administration agreed that only 10 nursing students would be assigned to each center. A relationship with a center in Brevard County already existed for the placement of RN-BSN students. It was decided to expand the involvement there for generic students as well.

To find other possible clinical neighborhoods, the Curriculum Revision

Coordinator and another faculty member discussed options, conducted windshield surveys, researched statistics regarding potential locations, and met with various community leaders to discuss possibilities. Care was taken to thoroughly research political climates of the partnership opportunities. No commitments were made until actual sites were agreed upon.

There was a desire to avoid partnerships with clinics associated with local hospital health care systems for two reasons. One reason was that these systems were changing configuration frequently and consistently, thus, the university did not want to get caught in one of these buy-outs. The second reason was that to align with one system might offend another, thus reducing additional clinical sites.

In all discussions the mutual expectations of and for the participant neighborhoods were determined. A legal agreement signed by appropriate administrators from each partnering group was given to all partners to place on file. An individual agreement exists for each CNC for provisions by the community partners such as disposable supplies, utilities, file cabinets, and telephones. The main tenets of the informal partnership agreements are as follows:

- The community's responsibility to the student includes provision of a safe site to practice and assistance with developing a relationship with the residents of the community.
- The university's responsibility is to provide consistent, on-going faculty and student representation within the neighborhood.
- The student's responsibility is to treat the residents of the community with respect, remain non-judgmental of the residents, and maintain confidentiality of information learned from the residents.

Desiring to initiate relationships with the residents, partnerships were formed with the Orange County School System; Central Florida Medical Clinic; Orange County Medical Clinic; Health and Community Services of Orange County; and Central Florida Area Health Education Center.

As faculty members grew to know more about "their" communities, indirect relationships developed, enabling further community initiatives within localities where CNC's existed. Eventually CNC's were developed in diverse areas of Orange, Seminole, and Brevard Counties. Populations served by the centers include Haitian, Puerto Rican, Cuban, Mexican, Jamaican, Black American, and poor southern Caucasian.

Criteria for selection of CNC Coordinators

UCF SON has 22 full-time faculty; 18 are assigned to the main campus in Orlando and four faculty members are assigned to satellite campuses. It

TABLE 3-2 School Of Nursing Course Design

Fall Semester: Year One	Total Credits—14
Focus: Healthy Communities and Healthy Families	
Health Assessment	3 cr
30 hr lecture 30 hr on-campus lab	
Therapeutic Interventions for Health Professionals	1 cr
30 hr on-campus lab	
Promoting Healthy Communities	3 cr
45 hr lecture	
Role and Function of Professional Nurse	1 cr
15 hr lecture	
Healthy Families across the Lifespan	3 cr
45 hr lecture	
Clinical Practice with Healthy Families across	
the Lifespan	3 cr
135 hr clinical	
Spring Semester: Year One	Total Credits—14
Focus: Promoting Physical and Mental Health	
Pathophysiology/Pharmacology	5cr
75 hr lecture	
Promoting Physical and Mental Health	5cr
75 hr lecture	
Clinical Practice in Promoting Physical and	
Mental Health	4 cr
180 hours clinical	
Summer Semester: between Year One/Two	Total Credits—6
Focus: Critical Examination of Nursing Practice	
Nursing Research	3 cr
45 hr lecture	
Elective	3 cr

(continued)

was decided that a specific faculty member would be assigned to each partnering community. Factors considered in considering faculty members for each CNC included:

- strong agreement with the new curriculum revision
- prior history in community health
- desire to work within the community health setting

TABLE 3-2 School Of Nursing Course Design *(continued)*

Fall Semester: Year Two	Total Credits—14
Focus: Acute Illness	
Nursing Care of Clients With Acute and	
Life Threatening Illness across Lifespan	4 cr
60 hr lecture	
Clinical Practice in Caring for Clients with	
Acute Illness	4 cr
180 hours clinical	
Leadership and Management	3 cr
45 hr lecture	
Nursing Intervention in Mental Illness	2 cr
30 hr lecture	
Clinical Practice with Mentally Ill Clients	1 cr
45 hr clinical	
Spring Semester: Year Two	Total Credits—14
Focus: Community as Continuum of Care	
Community as the Continuum of Care	3 cr
45 hr lecture	
Clinical Practice in Community-based	
Nursing Practice	2 cr
90 hr clinical	
Directed Practicum	4 cr
180 hr clinical	
Role Transition	2 cr
30 hr lecture	
Health Care Issues, Policy, and Economics	3 cr
45 hr lecture	

- desire to work with the particular population of the community
- distance from their home to the center (although this turned out to be a minor consideration)

Potential faculty members were then asked if they would be interested in a particular CNC and, if they agreed, the assignment would be finalized. The faculty member was then introduced as the CNC Coordinator to appropriate people within the neighborhood, and the relationship began. Once this occurred the Curriculum Revision Coordinator withdrew from any formal relationship with the neighborhood. This was done because it was believed that interacting with more than one faculty member could result in a confusion of information.

CNC COORDINATOR DEVELOPMENT

The Curriculum Coordinator conducted faculty development meetings. The first meeting was a luncheon meeting held in a lovely, quaint tearoom. Faculty members had time to get acquainted with each other in this new role. Their ability to support each other throughout this new adventure would be very important. At this meeting they were given notebooks with the vision, mission, conceptual framework, course syllabi, student assignments, and additional material. Subsequent meetings were held every other week as on-going development was taking place.

Each faculty member was responsible for researching the community for its patterns of formal and informal organization and becoming an active participant in its activities. Area Health Education Center (AHEC) grants provided summer salary for 40 hours for each CNC Coordinator so that they might continue the relationships formed within "their" community during the summertime when the students are not present. Each CNC Coordinator is scheduling their summer time in a different way. For example, one faculty member is continuing to take blood pressures at a senior center every other week, attend all community advisory meetings, and maintain communication with the school principal.

RESPONSIBILITIES TO THE STUDENTS

The CNC Coordinators are expected to assist the students in finding appropriate and meaningful ways of achieving their clinical objectives. They facilitate students evaluation of their Community Assessment, refer the students to specific groups within the community, and assist students in accessing key leaders in the community. The faculty assists students in determining strategies for gaining entrée into the community and with certain groups of residents. The faculty provides ongoing guidance for and evaluation of student activities.

RESPONSIBILITIES TO THE NEIGHBORHOOD

The CNC Coordinator is expected to:

- protect the community from unnecessary scrutiny by the students
- assure confidentiality of privileged information
- affirm that what is deemed important by the students is, in fact, important to the community

The CNC Coordinator is also expected to facilitate interventions that improve health care in their neighborhood by supervising students in provision of health promotion information and preventative screening activities.

Orientation of the students to their neighborhood

The students orientation begins with an overview of community nursing principles, a slide show with accompanying stories from a community health nurse, and a question and answer session. Students are then introduced to the CNC Coordinators for their assigned centers. From that point on, each CNC faculty and student group became responsible for meeting their own clinical objectives. As each neighborhood differs, the experiences differ; thus, objectives are met in differing ways.

Each CNC Coordinator meets with her students to began to form relationships with each other. Expectations of and for the students are explored. The directions to the center and the time for clinical experiences are given. Students are advised that they are expected to ride local transportation to the center the next day, which is their first clinical day. General information about riding public transportation is given along with instructions regarding things to observe along the route. Students are given time to discuss the specifics of where they would meet to begin their ride to their center the following day. Further orientation takes place once the students arrive at their assigned center.

At many centers it is possible to complete a "walk through" of the neighborhood. In other rural neighborhoods, a "drive through" is necessary as no sidewalks exist. Students began to describe their neighborhood from the "Windshield Survey" or "walking Windshield Survey." After assumptions are made from this exercise, information is validated by student's participation in a Key Informant Interview. Throughout the first semester, students from each center conduct a community assessment that results in a needs assessment to guide their activities throughout their remaining semesters in the nursing program.

RESPONSIBILITIES TO THE NEIGHBORHOOD

It is expected that students recognize that they are guests in the assigned neighborhood and that, as such, they:

- respect the residents of the community
- remain non-judgmental of the information of which they become aware
- maintain confidentiality with information of a sensitive nature

RESPONSIBILITIES TO THE COLLEGE

Students are expected to abide by the rules established by the university and the SON and documented in their university and SON Student Handbook.

Results of Neighborhood Partnerships

This community-based education program began in the fall of 1997, therefore, the assessment and evolution of these neighborhood partnerships continues. Each center is working at its own pace to accomplish goals designed for its specific neighborhood. Each community has identified the needs of the residents through its own assessment and continues to respond in identified areas. In addition, each center conducts or participates in at least one health fair per semester. Several centers have conducted numerous functions.

One center is established in a rural older community comprised of a large number of native Floridians. The elementary school principal requested that her facility be considered for a CNC since no health care provider or facility exists within 10 miles of the area, and the residents of the community "don't like to drive into town" for care. This center was initially for placement of RN-BSN bridge students and opened in the summer of 1998. The CNC Coordinator believed that the students should complete the following within the first semester:

- A written Community Assessment and needs identification to be presented to the principal and whomever else the students and CNC Coordinator consider appropriate
- One health promotion or disease prevention activity for the school
- One health promotion or disease prevention activity for the community

Lice is a major problem in the schools. Due to a lack of funds and access to other materials the school had been providing families with a mimeographed sheet containing outdated instructions on lice treatment. For the school health project the students developed a lice control poster and a two-color brochure. The school principal was very pleased when presented with the poster and 500 color brochures for distribution to the families.

For the community project the students planned a Health Fair in conjunction with the July 4 community festivities. Extensive brush fires in the area destroyed parts of the town so all festivities were cancelled. The students felt that they had made a commitment to this town and unanimously agreed to conduct the Health Fair at the Post Office when the town had returned to more normal condition. They returned after the end of the course to fulfill their assistance to the residents.

In addition to the Health Fair activities, the students presented material on safe drinking water. Safe water was assessed as an issue within this rural community since many residents have well water and numerous farm animals roaming on their land. Even those residents with town water are not immune to problems. During the time that the students were completing their assessment, some of the residents with city water were being instructed by the municipality to boil their water due to contamination.

Students assigned to a poor inner-city community consumed with crime and negative press selected families with the goal of helping improve their living conditions. One elderly woman was living in a filthy, unsafe house with poor flooring and broken furniture. She was homebound and had no consistent means of obtaining food or supplies. She would give money to buy food to her only relative, a young man with a drug habit. He would disappear for days and when he returned he would have neither money nor food. The students secured for the woman appropriate furnishings and flooring. In addition, they established a referral source for getting food delivered to the woman.

The health care needs of residents are being addressed through health fairs offering preventative services such as blood glucose monitoring and hypertension screening, information on breast and testicular examination, dental care, newborn immunizations, and self-administration of medications. One community had a history of residents not participating in health-related activities that were organized by local health care providers. When students chose to organize a health fair based on the community residents' survey results, more than 250 residents participated. When the community residents were given a voice to communicate their needs and concerns, the product was able to meet their needs and they participated.

Other health promotion and disease prevention activities include:

- Teaching classes:
  - Hygiene for Kindergarten, first, third and fifth grade
  - Safety education for fifth grade
  - Health education for sixth grade
  - Nutrition education at a Senior Center
  - Communicable disease prevention for the elderly
  - Reading food labels with elderly
- Delivery of meals for the homebound with Meals-on-Wheels
- Provision of weekly hypertension and blood glucose monitoring for elders at a Senior Center and at a Hot Meals Center
- Needs assessments of community nursery-child care settings

- Preschool and school-age screening
- Home visits for young childbearing and child rearing families to provide education about infant and child care and to identify high risk families
- Developing a referral system for teachers
- Weekly lice checks for whole classes of children
- Administering influenza injections (one group administered 450 injections)
- Participating in Health Start coordination and screenings
- Implementing dental health & hygiene project with after-school program participants
- Collaborating with a senior Assisted Living Facility to
  - Lead physical exercise activities
  - Implement pet therapy for the elderly

Longitudinal experiences

During their junior year, students initiate longitudinal projects within the community. In some instances, it takes at least two years for significant health care changes to occur. One student met a 71 year old woman (we will call Mrs. A) while riding with the Meals-on-Wheels program. Mrs. A was living in what could only be described as a "shack of a house" on a street in the Parramore area of Orlando. The student found that the woman was essentially immobile as she could not walk easily around the house without fear of falling through the rotted flooring. The toilet was "basically inoperable" so she sat on newspaper, placing the soiled ones in plastic bags until a neighbor came to remove the trash. The kitchen had no functioning appliances and there was no hot water. The house had no heat or air-conditioning, no screens, and rotting floors in every room. The house was visibly infested with roaches, mice, and rats.

The student returned many times to visit Mrs. A and take her vitals. She assessed that the woman had hypertension and "severe pitting edema" in her lower limbs. The woman had Humana PCA/Medicaid insurance and was entitled to care but had no way to get there. As the contact with the student continued, Mrs. A revealed that her Medicaid information card and number were available only at her landlord's medical office. Further exploration determined that the landlord (a doctor) was receiving Mrs. A's social security checks through the mail, requiring her to sign them over to him, then charging her $5 to cash the check. The landlord then deducted $325 for rent and another $125 for electricity, leaving Mrs. A with $25 for food and all other expenses for the rest of the month. The charge for the electricity seemed unjustifiably high since Mrs. A had one light bulb in the living room, one outlet in the living room, and one outlet for the refrigerator.

The student returned to the woman's home repeatedly trying to find ways to get help for her. "Social services made visits when I called them but nobody seemed to be able to relieve this kind lady of her miserable plight." When the student tried to get a visiting nurse service she was unsuccessful because Mrs. A did not have her insurance card or a doctor to order the visit.

After more than a year of working without success, the student decided to try a different tactic. She called in the Building Code Enforcement Department for help. Two inspectors responded to her insistent calls. One wanted to write the property up but his supervisor condemned the building. They then told Mrs. A that she had to be out in three days. The student asked if that meant three days not including the weekend. They said no that included the weekend.

Two hours later, the landlord appeared at the house yelling at a terrified Mrs. A. He screamed at Mrs. A for letting the inspectors in. He then stated that he had found another residence for her. The student asked the location of the new accommodations. She went to the site and on inspection found "there were three men living in the back on a mattress on the floor."

Returning to Mrs. A, the student found she "was experiencing chest, shoulder, and left arm pains." The student called 911 and Mrs. A was taken to the emergency room. The student explained to social services about the woman's homelessness coupled with her immobility, and she was admitted to Florida Hospital. As a result, when discharged, Mrs. A was placed in a new, total care facility. There she has made friends, sings at the church services, and says she "feels like she died and went to heaven."

Mrs. A lived for 5 years with the fear that if she complained she would be made homeless without recourse. She didn't know there were places like the one she is now in. It took this student time to first gain Mrs. A's trust. Then she investigated and advocated for her through a bureaucratic system, eventually releasing Mrs. A from the grip of her landlord. In effect, the student saved Mrs. A's life.

As successful as this case was, not all client problems can be cleared up within even a two-year time period. For that reason, as students prepare to graduate, the CNC Coordinator facilitates a meeting of juniors and seniors, and the senior students report on those needs or problems that they identified that have not been resolved. They are giving reports to the next shift so that identified needs or problems do not become forgotten.

SUMMARY

Between August 1996–1997, complete curriculum redesign and implementation occurred at the UCFSON. All faculty members actively participated in this process under the guidance of a Curriculum Coordinator. As a result all didactic and clinical courses are new. First semester students are introduced to the community as the framework for understanding the functioning of families and the epidemiological basis of health and health events. During the second semester, the students ntegrate a holistic model of nursing practice for individuals and families experiencing health risks, chronic health problems, or short-term illness with simultaneous concern for mental and physical health needs. The third semester focuses on the family that is no longer able to care for the individual or family at home where acute care is needed. In the final semester, students learn the role of a nurse as a change agent and case manager for health care. Working within a community-based practice model to effect changes in the health status, health risk and self-care capacity of target populations prepares students to practice in a variety of settings.

Since beginning the new curriculum, additional CNCs have been added in a migrant community, a low-cost government subsidized apartment complex, and an elementary school. Faculty has become strongly committed to this primary care, community-based curriculum. Students have expressed the desire to seek employment in a variety of acute and community settings. Most importantly, residents of medically underserved neighborhoods have benefited by the health promotion and preventative services provided by the UCFSON nursing students.

REFERENCES

American Association of Colleges of Nursing (AACN). (1997). *A Vision of Baccalaureate and Graduate Nursing Education: the Next Decade*. Washington, DC: Author.

National League of Nursing. (1998). *Visions II community-based nursing education project*. New York: Author.

Pew Health Professions Commission. (1991). *Healthy American: Practitioners for 2005: An agenda for action for health professions schools*. Durham, NC: Author.

Shea, C. (1995). "Laying the Groundwork for Curriculum Change." in P. Matteson (ed.). *Teaching Nursing in the Neighborhoods—The Northeastern University Model*. New York: Springer.

4

"Knocking on 99 Doors": The Experience of The College of New Rochelle (New York)

Marie Truglio-Londrigan, Joan Arnold, Marie Santiago,

Margot De Sevo, Mary Alice Higgins Donius,

Geraldine Valencia Go, and Anne Du Val Frost

"Knocking on 99 Doors" may sound to the reader like the title of a children's song but, to the College of New Rochelle School of Nursing, "Knocking on 99 Doors" is our designation of an effective strategy for engaging community residents in a partnership for the promotion of neighborhood health. Indeed, the experience gained from a class of senior nursing students who knocked on the doors of each and every resident of an apartment complex in Mount Vernon, New York helped to facilitate a curricular shift within the College of New Rochelle School of Nursing.

In 1998, a community health nursing group was assigned to a section of the city of Mt. Vernon, Westchester County, New York for its clinical rotation. On the first day of clinical, the students and faculty sought to learn about the neighborhood. To gather some basic information about the area, the students conducted an environmental survey of the four blocks of the neighborhood using their five senses. Students and faculty noted the surroundings and discussed the history of the neighborhood and the individuals who lived there.

During the walk, the students became interested in a new apartment building for older adults. It had been built in response to a need for affordable housing for the local elderly. After learning about the building's residents, the students identified a potential for the development and implementation of a community-based health promotion program at that site. A telephone call by a college faculty member to a known resident of the building served to begin the partnership process that would directly involve the students with the residents of the apartment complex and the surrounding neighborhood.

A meeting was held with the resident, the students, and the faculty member. The students asked many questions of the key informant and discovered that the building contained 99 apartments. Most of the residents were age 65 to 101 years old, the vast majority were of African American descent, and most lived alone. Although all residents were autonomous in self-care, most had one or more chronic health problems and were taking multiple medications to manage their illnesses.

The students expressed a desire to speak directly with the residents of the apartment building in the hopes of developing a meaningful, health promotion programs for the tenants. With the objective of working with the elderly as partners in care, the students held two, well-publicized focus groups the following week. Unfortunately, only six residents attended the group sessions. During the meetings, the elderly who did attend seemed shy and reluctant to participate.

The students were discouraged, not understanding why so few individuals participated despite their attempts to be inclusive. The faculty discussed the poor attendance and group dynamics with the students. After much brainstorming, the students realized that, although it would take more time and effort, they would have to try other strategies to gain the residents' confidence. Indeed, only the residents themselves knew about the health care needs of the neighborhood and how the students could help them.

The students concluded that the best way to reach out and establish trust with the residents was to engage in an action that would demonstrate caring and a willingness to take the extra step. With the key informant's blessing, the students proceeded to knock on every door within the apartment complex, introducing themselves and expressing their desire to work with the tenants to develop and implement health promotion programs. During the planning stage, the students initially expressed concern that the residents would not open their doors, but "Knocking on 99 Doors" proved to be an effective means of outreach. Not only were the residents willing to open their doors, surprisingly, they talked openly with the students, sharing concerns about themselves and contributing ideas for needed health education programs.

As students progressed from door to door, they documented the residents' concerns and suggestions. After compiling and reviewing the data, it became clear that, similar to the published demographics of the area, the residents' main health problem was hypertension.

A finding, unexpected by the students, was the discovery that many of the elderly felt overwhelmed by the stress in their lives and that they needed to learn ways to cope with the stress. The students had not been aware that stress would be an identified problem for older adults.

The residents also expressed concern about the medications they were taking, including a lack of basic knowledge about the medications themselves, administration procedures, and the medications' side effects. Additionally, the residents shared a discomfort with asking their primary health care providers for information about their medications. This lack of assertiveness resulted in an even greater confusion about their prescription regimens.

As the students went from door to door talking with the residents, suggestions about times for a health promotion program were obtained as well as ideas about the ways to best publicize the event. In response to the clients' input and needs, the students developed a health promotion program that was enthusiastically attended by 48 of the building's residents. The students provided the residents with needed information on medications via a culturally popular bingo gaming strategy MEDGO (Du Val Frost, 1995), cardiovascular disease risk factor appraisal and screening, and holistic modalities that they could use for stress management.

Without "Knocking on 99 Doors," the students and residents would never have become partners in the development of the meaningful project. Rather, the students would have been providers of care and the residents, if they participated, passive recipients.

Indeed, the students would never have identified stress management or medication management as needs of the population. More importantly, however, is the fact that many fewer of the residents would have even attended the health promotion workshop. By inviting the clients' active participation in the process, the students were able to garner a broad base of support among the residents as well as to meet the expressed needs of the group.

THE EMERGENCE OF A NEW MODEL: THE NEIGHBORHOOD-BASED CURRICULUM

Clinical competency is emphasized in the curriculum at the College of New Rochelle through its seven major theory/clinical courses. These courses are: Foundations for Nursing Practice, Adult Health I and Adult

Health II, Parent Child Nursing, Psychiatric Mental Health Nursing, Community Health Nursing, and Transition to Professional Practice and Leadership. Critical analysis is a highlight in the clinical application of theory and integration of cognitive, affective, and psychomotor learning.

Reviewing the Curriculum

The current curriculum of the school has always included community health concepts, with the experiences offered during the last semester of the senior year. In this course students have the opportunity to affiliate with home care and community health agencies. Their clinical experiences include home visiting of clients and collaborating with community health care agency personnel in implementing health promotion projects. Although the experiences have been extremely positive, both the faculty and students felt that there was heavy emphasis on assessment, diagnosis, and planning with minimal focus on intervention and evaluation.

The major deficiency identified by the faculty was the lack of integration of community concepts and experiences throughout the curriculum. Furthermore, except for the clinical experiences in the last senior level course, the majority of clinical experiences were in tertiary care settings with an emphasis on episodic care.

The faculty saw an urgent need to revise the current curriculum, not only as an academic exercise but also to enhance the community educational experiences of students who would soon be professional health care providers. An environmental scan, done as part of a strategic planning process for the curriculum, revealed a new focus in the current trends in health care delivery, the development of new educational models, increasing diversity of the student body entering nursing education, and a change in the populations they serve.

The most compelling trend in health care identified by faculty was the downsizing of acute care beds and the movement of care into the community. This movement was perceived as a positive one for the health care of all people in light of the challenges presented in Healthy People 2000: National Health Promotion and Disease Prevention Objectives.

Facilitation of Change

The faculty also identified strengths within the school that would facilitate the potential curricular changes. The school has a diverse student body, and this diversity is mirrored in the communities served. In addition, the students' curriculum has many positive aspects such as courses in transcultural nursing, course content, and experiences that prepare students to implement health promotion and a faculty increasingly committed to re-aligning the curriculum in order to prepare nurses competent to meet the health care needs of the people in their communities.

To begin the process of change, a faculty member was designated to explore different models of community-based education. She attended several workshops and had consultation sessions with the faculty of Northeastern University where a neighborhood-based nursing education curriculum had been implemented. An intensive workshop about this neighborhood-based curriculum provided by the faculty member excited her colleagues. A task force was formed to explore the feasibility of a new curriculum at the College of New Rochelle. The wheels for a new curriculum were set in motion.

The community-as-partner model (Anderson & McFarlane, 1996) was chosen to guide the implementation of community concepts across the curriculum. This model emphasizes the community-as-partner with a wheel design used to illustrate its core component and the eight subsystems. The core of the wheel represents the people who live in the community and their beliefs, history, and values. It is surrounded by eight subsystems including the physical environment, education, safety and transportation, politics and government, health and social services, communication, economics, and recreation (Fig. 4-1).

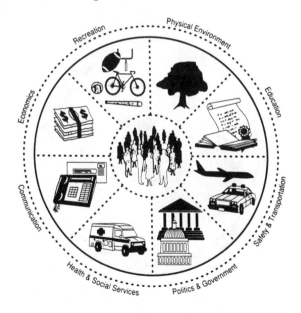

FIGURE 4-1 The Community Assessment Wheel. Community As Partner: Theory and Practice in Nursing. By Elizabeth T. Anderson & Judith M. McFarlane. Copyright 1996 by Lippincott-Raven Publishers.

Implementation of Change

Curricular change began with the focus in the first clinical course, Foundations for Nursing Practice. Students in this course addressed the first subsystem of the Anderson and McFarlane model, the physical environment. Subsequent clinical courses address the remaining seven subsystems.

To implement the curricular changes neighborhoods for clinical experiences were identified. Mount Vernon, New Rochelle, and Districts 10, 11, and 12 of the Bronx were selected because of their geographic proximity to the college and the diversity of the residents in those neighborhoods. Students were self-assigned to one of the identified neighborhoods and expected to return to that neighborhood for community clinical experiences.

When students enter their last clinical course, Transition to Professional Practice and Leadership, they have completed the assessment of all of the subsystems of their neighborhood. Thus, they are prepared to meet the needs of clients, family, and aggregates within the context of that neighborhood.

To further guide and assist the student to view community health from a broader perspective, the faculty implemented The Alliance for Health Model (Klainberg, Holzemer, Leonard, & Arnold, 1998). This model assists the students in understanding the interrelatedness of com-

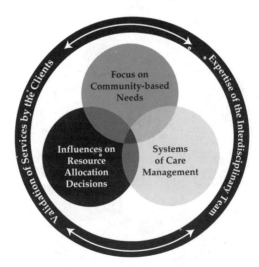

FIGURE 4-2 The Alliance for Health Model. Community Health Nursing: An Alliance for Health. By Marilyn Klainberg, Stephen Holzemer, Margaret Leonard & Joan Arnold. Copyright 1998 by The McGraw-Hill Companies, Inc.

munity-based needs, systems of care management, and the multitude of factors that influence resource allocation decisions within the context of the expertise of the interdisciplinary team and the validation of services by the client (Fig. 4-2).

As the process of implementing the new model slowly emerged, faculty and students were filled with a high degree of enthusiasm and sustained interest in improving clinical experiences that demonstrated their commitment to serving the diverse needs of the populations. Both saw the deeper development of roles of partners as critical to advancing health care in the neighborhoods.

PARTNERSHIPS FOR SUCCESS OF THE NEIGHBORHOOD-BASED CURRICULUM

There are four major partners in any neighborhood-based nursing curriculum model: (a) the people in the neighborhood, (b) the neighborhood's service providers, (c) the school's faculty with administrative support, and (d) students who establish and continue to maintain a relationship in a particular neighborhood. In this educational model each partner has essential roles.

Role of the Residents

The people in the neighborhood are individuals who identify the neighborhood as their place of residence. Demographic data would provide key elements of information about them, but an environmental survey is an excellent way to begin the acquaintance with the residents and initiate the establishment of a mutual relationship. The people in the neighborhood must initially be receptive to the purpose of the relationship and view it as a positive strategy that will benefit them. The role of the people in the neighborhood is to provide basic information related to health needs along with a willingness and capacity for change. This role means that they chose to contribute and provide input. It also means that each person serves as a conduit to other persons who might gain from participation. Additionally, the people serve as educated consumers of health services and programs and support programs by their active participation.

Role of the Service Providers

Service providers in the neighborhood have a dual role in relation to people in the neighborhood and the students. As service providers, they emphasize health promotion and disease prevention through their services and programs that address the needs of the people in that neighborhood. In this role they act as liaison between the people and students by facilitating the establishment and maintenance of working relationships. Their role with students includes facilitating clinical experiences, assisting and supporting students' needs for consultation, and directing students to available equipment, space, and supplies as necessary.

Role of the Faculty

The faculty provide the expertise regarding the educational experiences that will meet the needs of both the students and the people in the neighborhood. Their role is facilitator of the working relationships between the students and the service providers and the students and the people in the neighborhood. The faculty share, with service providers, information about students' level of knowledge and skills. This helps in planning and implementing health services and programs. The faculty also negotiate for clinical experiences that require the supervision of students by the personnel of the service agency. In addition, the faculty monitor all aspects of the clinical experiences as they relate to the school's curriculum and students' academic success.

Role of the Students

Students are the fourth partner in the neighborhood-based curriculum. Students bring their previous and current knowledge and skills to establish and maintain working relationships with the residents and service providers. Students collect comprehensive data about the neighborhood and the people through a variety of approaches. The process used in the initial encounter with the people in the neighborhood is critical in order to create a level of trust for further interactions and to determine the best strategies for future collaboration. Students share their successes and areas of concerns with the faculty and sometimes with service providers in an attempt to collaborate in accomplishing mutually decided goals. Students function as change agents and advocates for the neighborhood through their creative activities and projects that are based on the needs of the people. As students progress from one course to the next, they deepen their commitment to the people in the neighborhood and emerge as valuable human resources for the people. Students' impact on the neighborhood and its people can be so profound that they may, upon completion of their program, be asked to return as professional nurses of the service agency.

REFLECTIONS ON THE PROCESS

At this point in time, the development of partnerships with the people in the neighborhoods is taking on new meaning. In retrospect, this idea of "partnering with the people" seemed simple and easily accomplished. The process of writing this chapter, however, has required us to reflect on our progress to date. Our findings are enlightening and will be transformative.

We find that we have fallen into a trap! What we have done is to venture into the neighborhood, establishing partnerships with service providers while continuing our practice of nursing education as usual. The clinical experiences for students are the same with the exception of the location of experiences and the emphasis of community interventions.

One of our initial goals was to move to a community-driven curriculum, to an inclusion of our vision of how we care for and with a neighborhood by the actual engagement of all partners. We now realize that this cannot be accomplished by maintaining control and self-selecting what we believe to be the real issue: bombarding the neighborhoods with the educational programs, brochures, and videos as we believe appropriate (Bragg, 1997).

We now can see that we have just moved our experiences from one large tertiary building to a smaller neighborhood building. During the implementation process we have fallen prey to the concrete walls of the urban jungle, with the very doors designed to keep interlopers out proving to be effective.

Yet, the exemplar at the beginning of this chapter portrays how failure can inform participants and then, through creative partnering, lead to success. In that instance, we unknowingly stumbled into the essence of the neighborhood-based model. Care based on the needs of, and in partnership with, the residents is a different paradigm and the one we now seek.

LESSONS LEARNED

Unlocking The Secrets That Lie Within

It was humbling to learn that forming an authentic relationship with the people was the very essence of neighborhood-based nursing. The experience of truly being with a neighborhood proves instructive.

In our efforts at first, the neighborhood was viewed as a client in need of interventions to improve its overall health. The students were motivated to offer their expertise to shape these interventions based on their thoughtful assessments of the neighborhood. But the students were disappointed when their offers to provide service to address the diagnosed needs were not greeted with the same enthusiasm by the residents. It was not until the students truly listened to the residents about the neighborhood and its needs that the realization occurred.

Nursing in the neighborhood is based on the significance of an effective partnership with the residents. Once that base is secure, interventions are viewed as meaningful because they are truly responsive to identified needs. The secret of neighborhood-based care is effective partnering. The people are the center of the neighborhood. An authentic relationship with the residents as partners, along with the other partners in care, affords a mutual understanding of needs. Programs of intervention are greeted as responsive to residents' needs and the partnership idea is nourished.

Actions Speak Louder Than Words

The action of reaching out to the residents by knocking on their doors made it possible to learn directly through face-to-face interactions. The term "outreach" took on new meaning for the students as well as the residents. Instead of services being brought into a neighborhood, services were developed with the residents and tailored to their specifications. Needs were heard because students were ready to listen. Outreach is about making connections. The act of reaching out was perceived by the residents as an act of caring and experienced by the students as a caring action.

Nursing in the neighborhood and being with the residents fosters trust. Rather than caring for the residents, the students were caring with the residents. The ability to join with a neighborhood requires mutual trust and a commitment to stay with the process. This shift in presence occurred when the students decided to go directly into the neighborhood and knock on every door of the apartment complex. This act of "Knocking on 99 Doors" not only demonstrated the students' desire to hear what the residents had to say but also their commitment to work together to identify shared concerns and goals.

Shared Dialogue-Shared Understanding

Often, students carry out studies about the neighborhood from a distance, obtaining a peripheral understanding of the realities concerning residents about their environment. When people give voice to their description of their daily life experiences, they create a common ground for understanding (Shore & Freire, 1987). Once the residents opened their doors, the possibility of dialogue and understanding became a reality. The students' intention was to select a method that encouraged the capacity of the residents to voice their ideas, feelings, and beliefs. The students wanted to know what the residents thought, felt, and believed, and they wanted to find a way to work together.

The shared dialogue led to a shared understanding as residents in the apartment complex communicated their most pressing health needs and issues. Themes of concern became discernable and students were awakened to the residents' overwhelming concern about stress in their lives. The shared dialogue enabled the residents and students to plan and work together in a participatory change process.

The Power Within Us

Participatory partnership transforms health care transactions. When all partners assume responsibility and became actively engaged, there is the possibility of fulfilling a neighborhood's capacity for health (Kang, 1997). Health can not be transmitted by providers to residents, rather, it is achieved cooperatively through this mutual process.

The all too common fears about intruders and strangers that are evident when residents keep their doors closed were disappearing. Students were greeted by open doors. Some residents began to invest in the partnership by assisting in the preparations for Health Promotion Day. Some residents even supplied food for the event. The message was clear. Residents were saying: "Ask me and I will tell you" . . . "Include me and I will help you."

Through partnership building, the neighborhood's capacity for increasing positive health was enhanced. Residents chose to become active participants, thereby experiencing the power of intention. The residents knowingly were participating in the process of creating a healthier life and environment through their capacity to choose for health (Barrett, 1993).

FUTURE DIRECTIONS:
BUT OLD HABITS DIE HARD

The success of the nursing in the neighborhood curriculum is dependent on the relationships developed among the four primary partners of this educational model: the people, the service providers, the faculty, and the students. Although the faculty designing the curriculum had identified and valued these partners, the strategies for implementation of the model involved only three of the four partners.

Relationships among faculty, students, and service providers were already well-established, and it was easy to introduce new concepts for learning and practice with these groups. We spoke a common language and could develop common goals.

Relationships with the people, however, were not well-developed, and the ideas and opportunities for including them in the partnership were not well defined. Because of this, the key partner, the people, and a main objective of the model to enhance the health of the people through participatory change was all but lost.

The faculty came to the stark realization that the model for neighborhood nursing as we had constructed it was only being partially fulfilled. The faculty began an evaluation of the status of the program to determine the future direction of the curriculum. During the initial phase of this evaluation process, it became clear that a number of errors had occurred. In order for the curriculum to succeed, many difficult questions had to be asked and changes made based on the answers.

Identifying Neighborhoods

The initial question was: What is a neighborhood? At first, we had determined the neighborhoods by town lines and political boundaries. The five chosen "neighborhoods" were the city of New Rochelle, the city of Mount Vernon and three political districts in the Borough of the Bronx in New York City. We now realize that these areas simply are not neighborhoods. A neighborhood is defined by its people, not by city lines or political boundaries. Indeed, those who live on one side of Mount Vernon or New Rochelle may have little in common with those who live on the other side of either city. Similarly, the numbers of people who live in any of the three districts in the Bronx are enormous. A matter of a few blocks in any section of New York City can result in any number of changes, from ethnic make-up to types of buildings and businesses. A neighborhood is certain often diverse, but the important thing to keep in mind is that the people who live in the neighborhood have already determined where the boundaries lie and what they value. Formal boundaries do not create a neighborhood.

The faculty, therefore, are reevaluating the decision to choose Mt. Vernon, New Rochelle, and the sections of the Bronx as clinical neighborhoods. These five targeted communities, however, may still serve a purpose. Students may continue to collect assessment data and health statistics for these larger areas as a preliminary starting point. Within each of these larger communities exist multiple and diverse neighborhoods. Certainly, a number of neighborhoods must be chosen to accommodate the numbers of nursing students in the program, but a more critical eye will be used to identify these areas and their boundaries.

First, the areas should be diverse in population to provide the students with a rich, multicultural experience. Second, the neighborhood will include a health care facility that could provide the students with a base of operations throughout each clinical day. Third, the neighborhood may include a number of community service centers including houses of worship, schools, day care centers, food establishments, pharmacies, and other service and retail businesses. The faculty, therefore, must struggle with another fundamental question: Where are the neighborhoods? The answer to this question will only unfold over time as faculty commit themselves to this model by working within their communities. Exposure to the residents within the larger communities will make the entities of neighborhoods known to the faculty.

Establishing Partnerships

The next critical question for the faculty was: How are the partnerships made? During the initial phase of curriculum development for Nursing in the Neighborhood, a faculty member was responsible for contacting service providers in the designated neighborhoods in order to establish relationships and identify clinical placements. These service providers included nutrition centers, nursery schools, and senior centers. Although this approach seemed correct at the time, the faculty now realize that the way the community perspective was implemented continued to focus on experiences in episodic care. Merely changing the venue did not support nor integrate the concepts articulated in the neighborhood model.

A revised plan for the successful implementation of the neighborhood model is being developed. A full-time faculty member is assigned to each identified neighborhood. Ideally, the faculty member will spend at least one full day a week in the neighborhood developing relationships. Initially, the relationships will be with the service providers in the neighborhood. Knowledge of available services and existing educational programs is essential if the model is to be integrative and not episodic.

As partnerships are developed with service providers, key individuals in these organizations, as well as the neighborhood at large, will be identified. These key informants will be resources for faculty to come to know the neighborhood and to be accepted by the people of the neighborhood. The key people may be members of the clergy, or the hardware store owner, or the lady who lives in the third house on the left on Main Street. These key informants may have formal leadership positions in the neighborhood or may be average citizens who have assumed informal leadership through their actions. The key informants only become known by establishing a presence and trusting relationship with the members of the neighborhood.

No one accepts outsiders into their lives and homes without an introduction. Once relationships are made between and among the key leaders, the service providers, the students and the faculty, then the relationships will expand to include other residents and informal leaders of the neighborhood. This method of gradual introduction effectively facilitates the gradual incorporation of partners. It facilitates the introduction of the fourth major partner in the health care relationship, the people.

Curriculum Change

The faculty embraced the community-as-partner model (Anderson & McFarland, 1996) when Nursing in the Neighborhood was initially accepted as a concept. The model is clear, succinct, and inclusive of all the major factors that influence and impact a neighborhood. Unfortunately, as with any systems model, when it is divided into pieces it loses some of its essence. The question for the faculty is: How will the current curriculum integrate the Nursing in the Neighborhood model? The initial decision to maintain the curriculum structure was reaffirmed by the faculty. The challenge continues to be the successful implementation of the model given the existing structure.

Faculty discussions center on issues related to the specific learning experiences and student assignments needed to integrate and support the model. Since students are looking at discrete subsystems of the model in each clinical course, it was determined that course faculty are to assure that the pieces of the subsystem are continually viewed in relation to the whole model. If a student's learning experience requires moving beyond the subsystem addressed in a specific course in order to meet individual client or aggregate needs, faculty must plan, expedite, and mediate the opportunities for learning. By guiding the student to investigate other subsystems, the faculty supports both the student and client and maintains the integrity of the community-as-partner model.

Determining Student Assignments

Another question for faculty is: What should the student assignments be? As is often the case, faculty in the past made the assignments prescriptive and narrow. The nutrition center assignment in the Foundations for Nursing Practice clinical course, for example, forces the students to interview individual clients in relation to their dietary habits. Based on the completed assessments, referrals are made and a group teaching project is developed.

Using the Nursing in the Neighborhood as a framework for assessment, however, it is likely that nutrition is not the major need of the participants at the nutrition center. Clients may have a different value system related to food choices or have unexpressed concerns about the acquisition or preparation of that food.

A mutual process is just that—mutually inclusive of everyone, focusing on the group where needs and movement towards change comes from within, not from ideas, values, and beliefs that are externally imposed (Bragg, 1997). Within a partnership of care the clients are encouraged to participate in goal setting and the identification and development of the resources they need to meet those goals. Assessment and referral is a common process in health care, yet there is no mutuality to the process. There is no mechanism to learn about and assist with co-concerns in people's lives.

As illustrated in the exemplar at the beginning of this chapter, the residents in the building identified stress, blood pressure, and medication as their areas of interest. The possibilities of a population's needs are, of course, endless. The point is to identify the need of a specific neighborhood through dialogue with the people and to then develop an intervention with them.

Learning the Needs of the Neighborhood

There are many ways for the students to assess the needs of a neighborhood and develop programs with the people of the neighborhood, all while keeping in mind the goals of Healthy People 2005. Asking questions of the key informants and the people themselves is certainly one way. Another method is to make sensory observations of the neighborhood with extensive neighborhood assessments. Based on these assessments, the students and faculty may act as facilitators and mentors when proposing suggestions for programs that the people may accept or reject, participate in or ignore. As always, an informal dialogue with the people in the neighborhood will determine whether they feel a need for the identified program or whether their needs call for a higher priority.

Differentiating between Communication and Dialogue

As faculty continue to discuss the practical implementation strategies for the future of the neighborhood-based model, a theoretical question emerges: Is there a difference between communication and dialogue? Teaching students how to communicate with the people of the neighborhoods as they try to disseminate information is a strategy which is often neglected. Faculty spend hours discussing the individual nurse-client relationship, but how much time do faculty spend discussing strategies for communicating with neighborhoods and aggregates within those neighborhoods? Posters, billboards, bulletin boards, news print, radio announcements, and television spots are all techniques for communication with aggregates that faculty and students must know and use in order to communicate effectively.

Having identified the importance and value of the relationship among the four key partners, faculty automatically and without discussion assumed that the basis for these relationships was communication. Communication is essential for the exchange of ideas and messages. Dialogue, however, is necessary to come to a shared understanding. Therefore, the opportunity for dialogue is critical if participants are to be committed to the implementation of the neighborhood-based curriculum.

WHERE ARE WE NOW?

Participation and sharing must replace rigidity and defensiveness. Structured and unstructured dialogue among the faculty helps to crystallize the concepts, reveal and resolve dissonance, and generate creative implementation strategies. Perhaps the faculty jumped into a neighborhood-based curriculum endeavor with too much scattered energy.

At the present time, the faculty maintains continued interest and perseverance toward change. There are, however, the parallel emotions of confusion and, at times, fear. A commitment to the new and the unknown by virtue of its definition takes courage. Faculty who are leading curricular change need to serve as mentors and guides for those less comfortable in this change.

Meeting with small groups of faculty to discuss individual concerns helps to facilitate the process and will assist in the clarification of goals of the curriculum and to confirm support for the achievement of these goals. Curriculum change will not be successful without this dialogue. The dialogue requires a coming together to talk, to think, to question, and to challenge. This will move the process toward resolution with a shared understanding as to what neighborhood-based nursing can be (Bohm, 1992).

Students also need opportunities for a dialogue around the role of the professional nurse and the scope of future employment opportunities. We have started these discussions, however, there is need for further conversation to ensure that the students understand the reasons for the integration of Nursing in the Neighborhoods as the core of the curriculum rather than as an add-on to previous learning activities. Role socialization to the profession and to the neighborhood practice arena need to begin upon admission to the School of Nursing. The concept of a neighborhood may be introduced with an exploration of our college as the neighborhood. This process of data collection and knowledge development can then be applied to the external neighborhoods we serve in successive courses. Classroom teaching, case study work, examinations, and clinical experiences must integrate the expectations and experiences of a neighborhood focus.

Using journals and logs to articulate, analyze, and understand their experiences and perceptions enhances the student's knowledge of the neighborhood. These strategies also increase the student's reflection, sense of participation, and sharing in the process of becoming a nurse and a member of the neighborhood.

Bringing Neighborhood Providers into the Partnership

Dialogue with service providers is also critical if the theory of the neighborhood-based curriculum is to be supported by experiential learning. Although agencies are aware of the importance of community health care, there are questions yet to be answered: Are service providers ready to partner with the people within the neighborhoods? How will service providers respond to the people within the neighborhoods as they become more involved in this mutual process of building their neighborhood's capacity for health and realizing their own powerful potential?

If the business of health care is to be transformed from a hierarchical exclusive model to a model that supports the basic philosophical beliefs of openness, inclusion, and mutuality, then partnerships are necessary in order to provide learning opportunities which support the goals of the neighborhood-based curriculum. How can educators facilitate these partnerships? This is the challenge the faculty are beginning to examine.

Forming an advisory board inclusive of all the partners is certainly a possibility and one the faculty will discuss. Just as faculty have to be educated about neighborhood-based health care, however, so do all the partners in this endeavor. The School of Nursing must accept the challenge of exploring with the partners this new educational model, including what it means, how it is explicated, and what the possible outcomes may be.

The faculty believe the key to successful implementation of the neighborhood-based curriculum is dialogue. Dialogue is the glue that will form and solidify the partnerships among the significant stakeholders (Bohm, 1992). Shor and Freire (1987) noted, "Through dialogue, reflecting together on what we know and don't know, we can act critically to transform reality" (p. 99). What the faculty are seeking is a transformation in terms of how the partners think and act in order to promote the goals of Healthy People 2005 within their neighborhoods.

SUMMARY

In 1997, the faculty initiated the idea of curriculum change and started the process towards a Nursing in the Neighborhoods model. As with all transformation, success is more likely with periodic evaluation and reformulation. It surprised the faculty that, despite our commitment to the new model, our thinking did not easily change, and the curricular focus remained on content and not on the neighborhood. The faculty had all but left the neighbor out of the neighborhood. The process of inviting and expecting the residents to come to us was reversed when we reached out and the students started knocking on doors. Now we understand that we have only just begun the development of neighbor-to-neighbor relationship.

It is the intent of the faculty to revise the curriculum for greater emphasis on neighbor-to-neighbor strategies. Such strategies will be the focus of future dialogue. These dialogues will facilitate trust and increase mutual understanding of cultural beliefs. We will begin to understand the cultural basis for their beliefs, and they will begin to understand the culture of nursing education within which we function. This will then lead to developing strategies that are responsive to facilitating neighbor-to-neighbor health and ultimately the empowerment of the neighborhoods. The partners will begin the developmental process again, block by block, floor by floor, and door by door.

REFERENCES

Anderson, E. T., & McFarlane, J. M. (1996). *Community as partner: Theory and practice in nursing* (2nd ed.). New York: Lippincott.

Barrette, E. A. M. (1993). *Summary of the Barrette power theory.* Unpublished paper.

Ohm, D. (1992). *On Dialogue. Notice Sciences Review, 23,* 16–18.

Bract, N. (1999). *Health promotion at the community level: New advances.* Thousand Oaks, CA: Sage.

Brag, M. E. (1997). *An empowerment approach to community health education.* In B. W. Sparely, & J. A. Oleander (Eds.), Readings in community health nursing (pp. 504–510). New York: Lippincott.

Du Al Frost, A. (1995). *Cognitive theory.* In B. Schooner Johnson (Ed.), *Cognitive Theory* (pp. 89–97). New York: Lippincott.

Kang, R. (1997). *Building community capacity for health promotion: A challenge for public health nurses.* In B. W. Sparely, & J. A. Oleander (Eds.), *Readings in community health nursing* (pp. 221–231). New York: Lippincott.

Klainberg, M., Holzemer, S., Leonard, M., & Arnaud, J. (1998). *Community health nursing: An alliance for health.* New York: McGraw-Hill Nursing Core Series.

Shore, I., & Freer, P. (1987). *A pedagogy for liberation: Dialogues on transforming education.* South Haley, MA: Bergen & Gravy Publishers, Inc.

U.S. Department of health and Human Services. (1992). *Healthy people 2000: National health promotion and disease prevention objectives.* Boston: Jones and Barnett.

5

Moving Into Public Housing: The Experience at Winston-Salem State University (North Carolina)

Carol H. Boles and Sylvia A. Flack

On May 21, 1997, Winston-Salem State University's Nurse-Managed Center for the Elderly opened its doors in Sunrise Towers, a public housing development. One of the best known residents, Louise Davis, has lived in Sunrise Towers since it opened 28 years ago and serves on the Board of Commissioners for the Housing Authority of Winston-Salem.

At the Open House of the center, Ms. Davis explained to the local newspaper that "When we came in here 26 years ago, we were promised a nursing station and all the things that go with nursing." She is glad that the university and the housing authority finally figured out how to get nurses into the planned clinic space. As the university continues to develop this center, she is one of our greatest advocates.

Ironically, although Ms. Davis viewed the center as essential for her peers, she didn't think she needed the services herself. Being strong enough to sit through monthly board meetings, run the Resident's Council, and engage in many community activities, she often exclaimed to the center staff, "Listen, I'm in pretty good health."

One day when Carol, the Center director, was caring for Ms. Davis' neighbor, Ms. Davis asked Carol to check her blood pressure. It was found to be very high. Carol explored with Ms. Davis her diet and possible use of medications. Carol learned that Ms. Davis was using a homeopathic treatment in an attempt to control her blood pressure.

Further discussion revealed that several of Ms. Davis' family members had experienced strokes. After learning how hypertension contributes to strokes, Ms. Davis agreed to allow Carol to take her to the doctor and then to take a daily blood pressure medication.

Now Ms. Davis is not only a strong supporter of the center but also an active participant. In addition to regular blood pressure checks, she attends cholesterol screening and other laboratory testing sessions offered by the nursing and clinical laboratory science students. She has also joined the biweekly exercise class conducted by the physical education students.

Under the continuing care of the nursing students, Ms. Davis' blood pressure readings have been reduced and stabilized. She now participates in their educational programs addressing diet changes and other ways to stay healthy. In addition, Ms. Davis now serves as a case finder of other residents that need the assistance of students.

In addition to being a recipient of care, Ms. Davis also consults the students about the strengths and capabilities of people who are elderly. As president of the Sunrise Tower Residents' Council, Ms. Davis collaborates with the sociology students to plan programs for the residents. One of their most successful efforts was a Christmas celebration. During the development of the program LaCosta, one of the students, commented that Ms. Davis was insistent in wanting things done her way. Carol, the center director and LaCosta discussed the fact that Ms. Davis was the one who lived in and represented the community.

Carol referred LaCosta to a book, *The Careless Society and Its Counterfeits* by J. McKnight. In that work he explains that, when working for a community goal or vision, partnership with the community through individuals becomes the basic context for enabling people to contribute their gifts, (McKnight, 1995, p. 169). The student began to comprehend that, to develop successful interventions when working within a community of people, the individuals of the community must have the knowledge to assist the professionals and effectively accomplish their goals.

For the Christmas party the residents dressed up in their "glad rags," a term LaCosta had heard from her grandmother. The residents and students celebrated the coming of Christmas with laughter, singing, and fellowship. For weeks afterward, they talked about the activities and joy of the celebration. Programs such as this satisfy the human interaction needs so important to preventing social isolation and depression. The students recognize the importance of a party such as this Christmas celebration as a health promotion activity.

With Ms. Davis' ongoing leadership, the students have successfully planned and presented other programs for residents. Ms. Davis' expertise in the needs of herself and her neighbors is a valuable asset to the education of students and essential to the program of care in the center. Louise Davis offers just one example of how clients teach students how to be holistic, interactive, and responsive care providers.

PRIMARY CARE—DISEASE PREVENTION AND HEALTH PROMOTION

The Nurse-Managed Center for the Elderly is a primary care center with emphasis on health promotion and disease prevention for an underserved population. Through a reciprocal commitment between the Housing Authority of Winston-Salem and Winston-Salem State University, the elderly residents have received primary health care from the center staff, university faculty, and students. The disciplines of nursing, occupational therapy, clinical laboratory science, physical therapy, physical education, therapeutic recreation, and social science offer the primary care services.

Many of the elderly living in the public housing developments use the center as their primary care facility, the first contact when health problems occur or they have health concerns (ANA, 1987). Health services offered through the center include health assessment, diagnostic screening, health promotion education and activities, case management, skilled nursing care, and physician referrals as needed. Clients are also able to obtain social services counseling, occupational and recreational services, and physical therapy at the center.

The professional staff and students provide home visits for the individuals who are homebound. Residents are offered assistance with activities of daily living, including hygienic needs, nutritional services, and mobility assistance. They are also offered assistance with instrumental needs such as transportation, meal preparation, shopping, using the telephone, managing money, and performing routine housework (McEwen, 1998).

The National League for Nursing (1993) has taken the position that nursing education must shift to a community health care focus where health promotion and disease prevention programs are provided for individuals and communities. The Nurse-Managed Center for the Elderly is the ideal place to implement these community-based nursing learning experiences, not only in the community course but also in courses across the curriculum.

THE INTEGRATION OF CLINICAL EXPERIENCE WITHIN THE OVERALL PLAN OF STUDY

The Clinical Environment

A clinical experience in the Nurse-Managed Center for the Elderly focuses on integration of the course objectives with the residents' perception of their problem and needs. Obtaining the residents' input from the time of first identifying the problem through evaluating the outcome of the intervention is essential. Residents have insight into their circumstances and the greatest obstacles to their health. They also know their personal priorities. The learning process will not be beneficial for the student nor will the plan of care be effective unless it matches the residents' priorities and is seen by them as worthwhile.

Unlike the hospital setting, residents of Sunrise Towers live in the setting of care, and students are guests in this environment. This clinical environment is conducive to the application of theory to clinical problems, learning how to learn, developing skills in handling ambiguity, and becoming socialized into the profession.

The Student–Resident Relationship

Each of the 11 housing developments of the Housing Authority of Winston-Salem represents a unique neighborhood. Residents have a sense of ownership and pride in their own neighborhood. A respect of that ownership and pride is the first important attribute for success in the resident-student interaction. Students must realize that if the residents' perceive their attitude toward them as positive they will more likely welcome students into a collaborative effort to promote the residents' health. This resident-student partnership is essential for the success of the health promotion programs.

Critical Thinking

Before the students begin their clinical work, the director of the center confers with the students. The students learn that the care they provide is key to the outreach of the center. The framework for care is the students' ability to communicate with residents while combining assessment data with their nursing knowledge. Their success in health promotion and disease prevention activities depends on blending their critical thinking skills and care skills with the expectations of the residents and the policy and procedures of the center.

As an active agent in their learning process, the center offers the student an opportunity to utilize critical thinking through perceiving, questioning, and organizing facts and ideas and then shaping them into a meaningful frame of reference for action and problem-solving. An exemplar of how students learn to utilize critical thinking skills in this clinical experience is demonstrated through the experience of one junior nursing student.

During the Nursing of the Adult clinical experience, the student visited with one of the residents. During their discussion, the student and the resident identified several health problems. The student then discussed this list of problems and needs with her clinical instructor. One mutually agreed upon intervention was nutritional education to assist the resident in controlling her blood pressure. After gathering the essential data, the student used a computer to design an educational handout about the relationship between nutrition and hypertension. She then reviewed this colorful informational sheet with the resident and left it with her for ongoing referral.

The faculty member working with the student stated that, as she was creating the educational sheet, the student had smiled for the first time since being in clinical. The faculty member believes that this smile was brought on by the student's pride in being able to assist the resident and feel the gratification that comes from helping someone.

Student's Autonomy

Many students have commented that their clinical experiences in the Nurse-Managed Center provide the first insight that they have the ability to impact on the well-being of their clients. Working relatively autonomously with residents in their homes, students address a variety of health needs. This close collaboration provides students the opportunity for a more extensive assessment and development of a therapeutic relationship as they learn from the residents not only their concerns and needs but also how they feel they should be addressed. This process increases the opportunity for successful interventions. As Matteson (1995) noted, students in hospital-based clinical are usually not afforded the opportunity to practice with such autonomy.

Students in the RN to BSN completion program have the autonomy to decide how to meet their course objectives. Students employed in a local hospital choose to broaden their learning experiences through clinical assignments at the center. While working with these clients, they develop an understanding of the ability to function as autonomous providers in response to the reality of patients' lives. They learn from residents the critical importance of individualized discharge planning.

Two nurses decided to share this knowledge with the nurses with whom they work at the hospital at a monthly meeting of the hospital nursing staff. The students spoke with their colleagues about the knowledge gained from residents and how this neighborhood experience changed their nursing practice. Identifying the value of this new knowledge, developing a means to integrate it into their work in the hospital, and then sharing that knowledge with others in the hospital setting was a significant step in their growth as critical thinkers and their ability to affect change in patterns of practice.

Community Partnerships

Students find that the center's many community partnerships are essential in assisting residents with their health needs and provide opportunities for them to develop collaborative roles. McEwen defines collaboration as "the process of making decisions regarding health care management where individuals from various professions work with the client and the family or caregivers to jointly determine the course of care"(1998, p.17). Through the center, students collaborate with students and providers from a variety of disciplines as well as the residents.

As health providers, we frequently talk about the compliance or the non-compliance of the individual. Experienced students and faculty recognize that many residents are just unable to follow the health care plan that is prescribed for them. Residents have difficulty in identifying and contacting supportive community resources. At times, the processes are too complicated or exhausting for the elderly resident to easily succeed. This makes apparent the importance of an advocate in assisting the elderly to access the available community resources. It is not the will to be compliant that is missing but the means to be compliant that is the obstacle.

Students learn that they have the ability to bridge these obstacles for clients by collaborating with each other as well as a variety of community resources. Working with Crisis Control Ministry, an emergency assistance agency, students are able to help residents obtain medications when their finances and/or other resources were not adequate. When health screenings are needed, residents are referred to physicians in the local health centers. Students collaborate with the social service case managers when residents have questions about eligibility for financial assistance. Senior Services collaborates with students to obtain food, home health services, and special home care equipment for residents. When critical emergencies occur, the faculty and students work collaboratively with Emergency Medical Services and local emergency rooms.

Students find that Alexis de Tocqueville (as cited in McKnight, 1995) was correct in his description of a community. He believed that a community was a "small group of common citizens coming together to form organizations that solve problems." (p. 117). Students find that community organizations and services, such as the local churches and grocery stores, can help to solve problems experienced by this population.

By connecting the fragmented community pieces for the residents through collaborative partnerships, the students are able to meet the holistic needs of the residents.

Integration into the Didactic Classes

CASE MANAGEMENT

When a resident first seeks services from the staff of the Nurse Managed Center for the Elderly a chart is created. The data includes chronic and acute medical conditions, medications, nutritional habits, exercise and recreational activities, support systems, physicians, and the assigned social worker. These charts are kept on file at the center.

Many times it is the student who sees the resident for the first time and initiates the chart. Charts are available to students each time they come to the center to interact with the resident. With the guidance of the clinical instructor and the Center staff, the students update information and documents in the residents' charts. When students identify questionable or major changes as a result of a screening, i.e., EKG, the student and faculty contact the resident's physician and fax pertinent information to the physician's office.

A problem list and a list of screening results are kept at the front of the chart. This enables the students and faculty to follow up with the resident on identified problems and new treatments which the physician may have initiated. The student assumes the case manager role in interpreting the data into a plan of care. It is also the student's responsibility to communicate this plan to other members of the team.

PARTICIPATION IN RESEARCH

The research projects at the Nurse-Managed Center for the Elderly give the students an opportunity to participate in the research process. An essential principle which guides the selection of research projects for the center is that there must be a direct benefit to those who participate in the research.

During the PSA research project, the students were disturbed that this simple test was not readily available to the men in the community through Medicare. Many of the students had friends or relatives who had received an early diagnosis of prostate cancer through the PSA test for which their private insurance had paid. The students felt that this was a statement that, if you have money, your life and its quality is valued— if you don't have money your life is not valued.

One benefit of this research project was that students met and came to value the life of a poor person. Students were able to see the value of educating participants about the benefits as well as the negative issues of taking part in the research. Participating in the project also gave the student first hand experience of the need for being methodical in collecting the data from research participants as well as the importance of follow-up after the results of the test are completed. Without the assignment to the center, the undergraduate students would not have had opportunity to participate in a research project.

LEADERSHIP DEVELOPMENT

The development of leadership skills is facilitated in students as they develop health care responses to the needs of residents. In this setting the faculty or students may assume the leadership role when working with the residents and their support networks, other health care providers, local leaders, or the center staff. After identifying a need of residents, either on an individual or group basis, students take the initiative to seek the means to address that need.

Recognizing that residents have social needs that are often neglected, one of the nursing students planned a Thanksgiving celebration for the residents of Sunrise Towers. She took the lead in organizing the event and in soliciting the members of her sorority to provide the means of offering the residents a Thanksgiving celebration. Understanding that health promotion is more than ensuring that a client has food, she made it a holiday celebration that met the social and celebratory needs that promote mental health.

A student in sociology worked with the residents to plan a Black History celebration. The program included children from a local elementary school who sang and presented a play about the Black History of Old Salem. The main speaker was a 90-year-old resident who had grown up in the local area, attended The Slater Institute (forerunner of Winston-Salem State University), and had worked as a schoolteacher. Sharing her experiences, she described how life had been and how many important things in life have not changed. This student recognized the importance of sense of culture, inter-generational sharing and self-pride as well as pride in one's roots.

ECONOMICS OF HEALTH CARE

Through their interactions with residents, students become aware of the economics of health care from the consumer's point of view. Students are surprised that many of the basic needs that are vital for health such as food, cleanliness needs, resources for basic activities of daily living, and access health care are difficult to obtain when living on a limited income. As students advocate and seek care for residents it soon becomes obvious to them that Medicare is helpful when one is in the hospital, but not for the daily management of chronic diseases. Students also learn about the limits of eligibility for Medicaid as some of their clients miss being able to participate in that program because their income is $15 to $20 too high, even though they have $50 to $500 worth of medication bills. Students' perceptions that health insurance and government programs enable the elderly to easily acquire the means to maintain their health is replaced with the reality that individuals sometimes have to make choices between food and medication.

NEIGHBORHOOD-BASED NURSING EDUCATION

The Neighborhood

The Winston-Salem State University's Nurse-Managed Center for the Elderly is located in a high-rise called Sunrise Towers in East Winston-Salem. This public housing development is managed by the Housing Authority of Winston-Salem and is located in an area with a number of public housing developments.

Historically, this has been an African-American neighborhood. More recently, a large number of Hispanics and European Americans have migrated to this area. There is a church within walking distance of almost every development.

The neighborhood is a mixture of factories, modern homes, ghetto areas, public schools, and commercial businesses. Many "mom and pop" stores are no longer in business.

Health care providers to the area are the local health department, the Reynolds Health Center, and the Centerpoint Mental Health Center. Two major medical centers, Wake Forest University Baptist Medical Center and Novant Health, are located in Winston-Salem and offer services to this population through outreach clinics. Although these facilities are geographically close to the elderly, transportation and mobility problems make it difficult for them to access services.

Winston-Salem State University is located within the same neighborhood and educates a number of health care providers. The faculty of the Division of Health Sciences, through the Nurse Managed Center for the Elderly, offers primary (preventative) care to geriatric residents in the public housing developments. The center, managed by a professional nursing staff and under the auspices of the university, operates as a multidisciplinary organization. Services are offered through the departments of nursing, clinical laboratory science, occupational therapy, physical therapy, social science, physical education, and therapeutic recreation.

Educational Partnerships

The center was created to provide care for elderly residents and a clinical learning site for students. The Steering Committee and the Advisory Board for the center have been instrumental in developing this educational partnership.

The Steering Committee is composed of the Winston-Salem State University Department Chairs of the departments who participate in the center and some of the Housing Authority managers. The purpose of the Steering Committee is to serve as the governing body of the center. The department chairs were placed on the committee in order to enhance the educational function of the center.

The Advisory Committee is composed of university faculty, elderly residents, health care professionals, community agency representatives, community residents, county and state officials, and Housing Authority personnel. They keep the center staff informed of any community changes that may effect the center's operations and the feasibility of educational experiences for students.

The center was designed to provide health care in the area of health promotion and disease prevention. The faculty and students provide care for the residents as part of their clinical educational experience, with the department of Nursing the largest provider of care.

ROLE OF THE STUDENTS

The nursing students' first clinical experience at the center begins in the Assessment of Health Alteration Course. They develop their health assessment skills by assessing the health status of the elderly residents. In addition, students develop their foundational nursing skills and develop competency in utilizing the nursing process through their experiences with center residents.

Additional interactions with the residents occur in other courses. Each student in Gerontological Nursing adopts a resident as a grandparent. Students in the Adult Nursing courses at both the junior and senior level manage the care of residents who have acute illnesses and complex chronic disease. The nursing students in Community Health Nursing focus on the elderly population as part of the community. Their emphasis is on meeting the health needs of elderly clients living in this environment. The students in Mental Health Nursing also come to the center to exercise the nursing roles of caregiver, teacher, counselor and client advocate.

Other university departments that provide student experiences in the center include Clinical Laboratory Science, Physical Education, Sociology,

Occupational Therapy, Therapeutic Recreation, and Physical Therapy. Some of these educational experiences are interdisciplinary in nature.

ROLE OF THE RESIDENTS

To be eligible to participate in the activities of the center, clients must be 62 or over and live in a residence of the Housing Authority of Winston-Salem. The residents are partners in identifying needs, exploring potential resources, and determining the services of the center. They also keep abreast of activities offered within the community by other organizations that will benefit all residents.

One of the residents informed the center staff that the Salvation Army was giving out Christmas boxes of food, however, they required individuals to come to their facility to register for the boxes. After checking with the Salvation Army, the center staff transported 40 residents to the Salvation Army building in university vans.

To accommodate the residents who were unable to ride in the van, the Salvation Army allowed the center staff to assist the residents in completing their applications at the center. Eighty-seven residents registered. After the registrations were completed, each resident was then required to pick up the box from the Salvation Army. Because of transportation problems, the Salvation Army allowed the center's staff to pick up all the boxes and distribute them from the center. This is just one example of how a resident initiated an effort which lead to collaboration between community agencies and resulted in a benefit for many in the neighborhood.

ROLE OF FACULTY

After a review of the curriculum, the faculty determined which course objectives could be met through clinical experiences in the center. All faculty involved in the selected courses are oriented to the center. Using their skills in creative problem-solving, faculty help students meet the holistic health needs of the residents. Faculty who are interested in developing innovative community outreach programs are most successful in developing learning experiences in the center for students.

Bridges Created between Faculty and Neighborhood

Faculty members with a broad interest in the clients of the center are able to develop partnerships between the center, its residents, and the community. One example was a faculty member who asked the Women's

Missionary Society of her church to provide their community service in the center. The church is located across the street from one of the developments and many of the residents are members of the church. The missionary group sent food and personal care items to be distributed to the residents.

Faculty-Developing Partnerships with Nursing Agencies

Developing partnerships with local home nursing agencies has been essential in the collaborative care of the residents. Some of the residents have routine visits by a nurse from a home health agency. One faculty member who has established her faculty practice in a home health agency took care of a neighborhood resident who was on a ventilator. While working with this resident, she asked her if she would like for student nurses to help with her care. The resident agreed. When the faculty member came to the center with her clinical group, caring for this resident was included as one of their experiences. The students, the center, the home health agency, and the resident benefited by this faculty's connection to each of them.

When faculty practices are connected with agencies, this enhances the nursing agency's respect for the skills of faculty and their students. When the faculty practice is local, it provides the opportunity for developing joint ventures of care. This results in a stronger collaborative effort in meeting the health needs of the homebound resident.

Faculty Responsibility to Students

Faculty members facilitate students' mastery of learning objectives in this innovative clinical area. Students learn the appropriate nursing skills, and offering them the opportunity to work with aged residents in the community fosters the development of positive attitudes toward the elderly. The pre- and post-attitudinal surveys of our students indicate a significantly positive change in their attitude toward the elderly.

Faculty members also facilitate research and the collaborative efforts within a multidisciplinary team. One of these multidisciplinary efforts was a Prostate-Specific Antigen (PSA) blood screening research project. The nursing students prepared and presented educational sessions for the residents about prostate cancer. The presentation included the pros and cons of having a PSA screening. The sociology student researched the availability of the PSA test for men in the underserved community and found that Medicare did not pay for the initial test.

Clinical laboratory students research the validity of the test and found that the PSA test validity is higher than the manual exam for which

Medicare pays. Nursing students reviewed the consent forms with the participants prior to the test. Students from the clinical laboratory science students drew the blood samples for the PSA test. There were three positive PSA results from the screening of 21 men. The center staff ensured that these individuals had follow-up visits by their physicians. Through this experience, students were able to see the strength of working together in a multidisciplinary team.

Faculty Responsibility to the Resident

Maintaining the dignity of the residents is a high priority of the staff, faculty, and students at the center. One of the premises for establishing the center was that underserved individuals do not seek health care because many health care providers are culturally insensitive. Faculty and staff work with along with the students in providing culturally sensitive care to the residents. The importance of respecting and incorporating the values of the residents is taught and reinforced through the role modeling by the faculty and staff.

"Cultural values are principles or standards that members of a cultural group share in common. Values serve several important functions ... they serve as a basis for attitudes, beliefs, and behaviors ... they help to guide actions and decisions ...they reflect a person's identity and (they) provide a basis for self-evaluation" (Luckman, 1999, p. 24). To successfully help the resident to live a healthier life, the provider must consider the foundational values of the residents when developing programs. Seeking the residents' input regarding their needs and seeking the residents' permission for the faculty and students to be involved in their lives is the foundation of the center's health promotion programs. Collaboration between the residents and the center becomes the framework in promoting the residents' health.

NURSING STUDENTS IN THE NEIGHBORHOOD

Criteria for Selection of Students

Students are selected through course enrollment and an expressed interest. During the students' first experience in the center, they tour the center and the neighborhood. Orientation includes handouts, which explain the operation of the center and the basic details of the documentation required by the center. The center is a subsidiary of Winston-Salem State University and belongs to the students and faculty. It is stressed to the stu-

dents that, since the center is part of Winston-Salem State University, faculty and students are professional representatives of the university in the neighborhood. It is also stressed to the students that, unlike the hospital setting, resources within the center are designed to specifically enhance the students' ability to care for the residents.

Student Orientation to the Neighborhood

The center is located in Sunrise Towers, one of the developments of public housing. All resident records are kept there. Clinical experiences take place in Sunrise Towers as well as the other 10 neighborhood developments of the Housing Authority of Winston-Salem.

Students initially conduct the "Environmental Survey" (Matteson, 1995, p.195). The environmental survey requires that the student tour the neighborhood. After touring the neighborhood the students' surveys include comments such as: ". . . a good place for residents . . . I felt comfortable, I had no fear because I felt these residents are good people. . . . The residents seem very nice and friendly . . . the residents were very friendly and helpful which helped me feel more at ease and at home." As students become involved in the care of the residents, they begin to see other aspects of the neighborhood that are not so desirable.

Student Responsibilities to the Neighborhood

Students are assigned to work with several residents. They phone the residents, visit them in their apartments, or see them in the center or in the common areas of the Housing development. As students work with residents, the realization that they have the same desires and problems as younger people surprises the students. Observing that the elderly may have sexual partners, that some have problems with money, and that some have problems with substance abuse is an eye-opener.

Students may have observed elderly in institutional settings being treated as children. In the resident's home, however, the students are quickly taught by their clients that they are in charge in their own home. The students learn to be respectful of the residents and respect their contributions.

As the students gain the confidence of the elderly residents, the importance of maintaining privacy and confidentiality becomes a priority. The philosophy stressed in the center makes it clear to the students that the residents' well-being and autonomous rights are of top priority, and confidentiality is an expected right of the residents.

NEIGHBORHOOD NEEDS MET BY THE STUDENTS

Students greatly enhance the center's ability to provide care within the neighborhood. During each semester, approximately 200 nursing students work with residents in the neighborhood. Each student partners with an individual resident to identify his or her needs, develop possible interventions, and consider desired outcomes. Students then discuss these findings with their clinical instructor. Together, the student and faculty review possible community resources that will help the resident accomplish the desired outcomes. After obtaining the approval of the resident, the appropriate community resources are contacted to assist in the resolving the resident's problem.

In their work students discovered that one resident had multiple health problems and limited resources with which to resolve these concerns. The problems included obtaining and using medication, assistance in cleaning her apartment, and the scheduling of physician appointments as well as transportation to the appointment, the need for participating in an AIDS support group, and financial assistance with her rent. These problems were addressed through the effort of students, faculty and the center staff interacting with multiple community agencies.

This holistic approach pieced together fragmented resources in order to resolve the resident's health needs. The students were relieved that these problems were attended to. Continuous evaluation and follow-up by the center's staff are now necessary to be sure that the solution stays intact. If any part of the support system ceases to exist, it will become necessary to seek other solutions.

Student's Longitudinal Experiences in the Neighborhood

Nursing students have clinical experience at the center during their sophomore, junior and senior courses (see Table 5-1). As students progress through the curriculum, they develop a clearer concept of nursing in the community and provide care to a series of clients. The center staff believes that students would receive additional benefit by following a group of clients through the progression of courses. This has not been incorporated into the faculty's plan at this time.

As students expand their own knowledge base of neighborhood residents' health care needs, they have the opportunity to develop more creative ways of promoting health and preventing disease or the progression of disease. The center staff has observed that students' clinical application has been enhanced when one faculty member is responsible for the clinical experiences of all students in each course.

TABLE 5-1: Winston-Salem State University
University/Community Wellness Center
Nurse-Managed Center for the Elderly

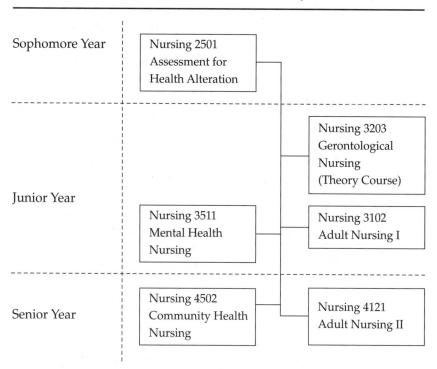

EVALUATION OF THE NEIGHBORHOOD-BASED CLINICAL EXPERIENCE BENEFIT FOR THE RESIDENT

Client Satisfaction

Through word of mouth the center has become well-known throughout the neighborhoods. More than 395 residents have received assistance from the center. Of the residents who completed the Pace University's Satisfaction Survey (Lienhard, 1992), all indicated that they would continue to use the center as a source of health care. Comments included "It's great! I feel that as long as Jesus is with you everything will work out fine"; "It is wonderful that the center is here to help take care of us"; "I appreciate the center checking on us and taking us to the physician, if necessary"; and "Very thankful that the center is here."

DATA COLLECTION

Both qualitative and quantitative data are used to evaluate the center's services. The center's external evaluation process, conducted by The Community Care Coordination Network (CCCN), includes pre- and post-program surveys of residents' health status and their use of community health services i.e., hospital, emergency room, and health clinics. These surveys are administered to residents in Sunrise Towers and in the other neighborhoods in an attempt to assess the benefits of the center's services.

Multiple scenarios have been documented in which health screenings by the center have revealed impending problems. In these situations residents were assisted in obtaining the assistance they needed and problems have been resolved before they became more severe. These documented scenarios have been used to evaluate the center's desired outcome of increased access to health promotion and health care.

The residents who live in Sunrise Towers, the housing complex where the center is located, frequently express their gratitude for the ease of access. One 90-year-old resident who came for assistance stated that it is so difficult as one gets older to even go to places where help is available. She also explained that, when you are hard of hearing, the telephone consultations are difficult and confusing. This confusion is increased when the recorded message goes on and on from one selection to another. She stated that the ease of access of the center was a blessing.

Several of the residents have had ongoing problems with their blood pressure. The center's location makes it possible for residents to have daily blood pressure screenings. If the readings are altered, this allows immediate discussion with the resident about possible causes. The cause could be diet, the fact that medication was not taken properly, or a stressful situation. These screenings enable the resident or the staff to contact the physician for follow-up if needed, or at least document the resident's blood pressure reading or other findings.

Accessing the health care system is cumbersome. At times, many different contacts must be made to even obtain an appropriate appointment. With today's time saving technology, i.e., the recorded phone directions, compounded with the residents difficulty hearing, lack of understanding of the terminology, and lack of energy or patience, the elderly are often unsuccessful. The center's staff, faculty, and students are able to make these appointments for the resident.

After securing the appointment, reminders are created to help the resident remember the appointment. Since the majority of the residents do not have transportation the center contacts Transaid, a local transportation system, to schedule the resident's trip to the doctor. If Transaid has no available space, someone at the center will take the resident to the doctor.

The residents who live in the public housing of the Housing Authority of Winston-Salem have limited financial resources. By the middle of the month, they frequently do not even have money for food. This means that, if the physician orders medication, there is no money to pay for it. In this situation, someone from the center may talk with the physician about possible drug samples. If this is not possible, other community agencies such as Crisis Control are called for assistance with the pharmaceutical needs of the resident.

It is the center's philosophy to do everything possible to help the residents be independent and self-sufficient. At times, it is necessary for the student, faculty, and staff to be the surrogate support system for residents. This may mean that the student, the faculty, or the staff member will pull out the mop bucket and cleaning supplies to clean the resident's apartment. It may also mean that food from the center's food cupboard is given to a resident.

Many times transportation is furnished for just an individual. At other times, a group of residents will have transportation needs. The exercise classes held biweekly by the physical education students involve transporting residents from three other complexes to Sunrise Towers.

One time, a resident expressed the desire for a group trip to the local drive-through Tanglewood Christmas Light Exhibition. The center staff makes a special effort to listen when residents identify a need or desire and request assistance. By responding in a positive manner, the providers indicate to the resident(s) that their thoughts are valid and valuable. When the residents believe they are valued, their participation in the program becomes more integrated.

Residents' evaluations of dinners, parties, and celebrations have been offered both verbally and in writing. The first Thanksgiving dinner, organized and paid for by the students, had a few glitches when 125 people showed up for the planned 100 dinners. More food was obtained, but the process of feeding the unexpected 25 was delayed. A few of the residents complained about the lack of food and how slow the service was, but none complained about the program or food. Many other residents expressed appreciation for the meal. Some of the students were resentful of the criticism and spoke among themselves saying that the residents should have been thankful for what was there.

The next Thanksgiving the students decided to plan for 175 for the Thanksgiving meal. The Zeta Phi Beta Sorority was approached to finance this Thanksgiving meal as a community service project. That year there was plenty of food to go around and the service was very prompt. Residents coming to the center office the next day expressed how grateful they were for the meal. Some of the residents wrote thank you notes and some even sent students Christmas cards thanking them for the dinner.

The senior citizens here have generally been very grateful for programs and services but, at the same time, have not hesitated to inform the center if they think they have a better way of doing things. Their input has been a valuable asset which has added depth and warmth to the center's programs.

ADVOCACY

The center's staff, faculty, and students often become a resident's advocate. The success of this advocacy is measured by outcomes. As an example, one resident came to the center requesting financial assistance for medications. He was specifically inquiring if he could receive medication from Medicare like his friend received. Further discussion revealed that his friend's medication assistance was through Medicaid. The man seeking assistance worked part-time and earned about $20 too much to qualify for assistance, yet monthly medication bills were over $200. He was quite adamant about not working any less than he did. Further discussion revealed that he was a veteran and should qualify for free medications from the Veterans Administration (VA). He chose to seek this assistance on his own and was given the name and phone number of the advocate for veterans. He now receives his medications from the VA and the staff at the center feel that they have been successful in advocating for him. He has maintained his self-worth by working as much as he is able and is receiving assistance that he earned through his service to his country. An advocate provides the best care by allowing and encouraging each resident to do what he believes is best and to be as independent as possible.

EVALUATION OF THE NEIGHBORHOOD-BASED CLINICAL EXPERIENCE BENEFITS TO STUDENT LEARNING

Exemplar of Critical Thinking Skills

Students are observed to see if they demonstrate characteristics of critical thinkers during their clinical experience at the center. Alfaro-LeFevre (1999) identifies critical thinking characteristics as: (1) criticism for the sake of improvement, new ideas, and doing things in the best interest of the key players involved; (2) inquisitiveness about intent, facts, and reasons behind ideas or actions; (3) thought- and knowledge-oriented, (4) sensitive to the powerful influence of emotions but focused on making decisions based on facts and what's morally and ethically the right thing to do; and (5) thinking independently unless dealing with complex issues or a situation too risky to approach with limited knowledge.

One student who was looking for the resident to whom she had been assigned knocked at an apartment door. The resident invited the student to come into his apartment. The student's first impression, as she sat down and talked with the resident, was how empty the apartment appeared. The man mentioned that he was a diabetic and had a hard time keeping his blood sugars at the appropriate level. He stressed that eating the right foods was one of his problems.

As the conversation continued, the student realized that this resident had not sought services from the center even though he had a need for assistance. She had knocked on the wrong door. Consultations ensued with her clinical instructor and the center director about working with this resident. It was decided that she could continue.

The student stated that the man seemed initially hesitant to talk with her, but gradually began sharing information. The student recognized that the resident was the key player in this situation, a key player who had needs that he was not meeting on his own.

When she made a return visit, he again invited her into his apartment. She screened his blood sugars and the reading was 50. The client stated that he felt fine. Further questioning did not reveal any acute problems related to the hypoglycemia.

Physical assessment revealed signs of poor skin turgor, protruding ribs, and a very thin stature. The man stated that he ate at McDonalds across the street most of the time. At this point, the resident indicated that it was time for the student to leave. The student arranged a time to visit the again the next day.

The student was very inquisitive about intent, facts, and reasons behind this man's not making an effort to meet his nutritional needs. This could be detrimental to his well-being especially since he had diabetes. That evening, the student thought a great deal about this resident. She knew the facts about how diabetes affects the body and the interventions that help the body compensate for the process of diabetes. She also recognized that this resident had other important issues that were a factor in his health status. She remembered the pride and independence that this resident displayed when she had talked with him. She wondered how she could identify the underlying problems while she maintaining his self-respect.

The next day, she visited the resident as scheduled. She wanted to just open the doors and see what food he actually had in his cabinets and refrigerator. She knew, however, she must maintain his self-respect; this was his home. She thought about what was morally and ethically the right thing to do. She decided to ask for his permission to look, which he gave. When she opened the cabinets and the refrigerator, they were empty.

This man felt the concern this student had for him and began talking. He told her what a difficult time he had in budgeting his money to obtain food and the other necessary goods throughout the month. He asked the student to help him.

She began by discussing the support system and financial resources that he had available. He received his Social Security check at the beginning of each month. None of his family visited or helped him in any way. He socialized with some of the neighbors, but they did not provide the support system he needed to promote his health. She assured him that she would try to find some resources to help him.

To this point she had thought independently, but she knew this resident's situation was too complex to address with her limited knowledge. She sought the input of her clinical instructor and the center director.

The student's interactions with the resident, clinical instructor, and center director lead her to the conclusion that this resident had the potential to be successful with health promotion efforts if he had the appropriate support resources. With their guidance she began accessing identified community resources for food and for an individual who was a reputable payee. She then made connection between the community resources and the resident. The next week she was back in the setting evaluating and fine-tuning the constructed support system for the resident.

This student meets the definition of a critical thinker (Alfaro-LeFevre, 1999). She was an independent and active thinker, open-minded, empathetic, curious, insightful, persistent, and a good communicator. The student was honest with herself and the resident about her skill level. The solutions she developed were proactive, organized, systematic, flexible, and realistic. She demonstrated that she was a team player by including the wishes of the resident and following the leads of the faculty and the director of the center while being creative and committed to excellence. This scenario is descriptive of the way the Nurse-Managed Center provides opportunities for students to demonstrate critical thinking skills. The other outcome from this educational process was to provide a flexible setting where students can gain autonomy as they design interventions which meet the holistic needs of the resident.

Evaluation by an External Organization

The Community Care Coordination Network (CCCN) is part of an external evaluation process to determine if the center accomplishes its desired outcomes. Students participate in gathering data through functional surveys. This gives them an opportunity to work with a research instrument to systematically collect data for entry into a database. Prior to conducting the surveys, the process of data collection and the survey instrument are reviewed. Demonstrations show students how questions should and should not be presented to residents. The importance of showing respect for the participants at all times is stressed.

Students learn through conducting this survey how difficult it is to get information from residents even though they have agreed to participate. The students often blame this reluctance to talk as inadequacy on the part of the center to properly organize and prepare the residents. They learn through discussion and experience that, in reality, the inability to easily obtain information from residents is related to the issue of trust and is only overcome through repeated interactions.

EVALUATION OF THE NEIGHBORHOOD-BASED CLINICAL EXPERIENCE BENEFIT TO THE NURSING FACULTY

Teaching nursing in the Housing Authority of Winston-Salem communities provides a setting which can stimulate the creativity and ingenuity of the nursing educator. The success of the educational process is evaluated by documentation of innovative experiences the faculty provides collaboratively with the students. One of the faculty members designed the Assessment for Health Alteration Course to incorporate assessment of the elderly in the center as part of the laboratory component. This enables students to assess individuals with chronic diseases in addition to assessing healthy peers. Looking at possibilities rather than trying to maintain status quo is essential for faculty to successfully teach students in the community setting. The faculty are valued for their input in program assessment and development, their evaluation of the learning experiences, and the response of both the students and the residents to the care.

Participating in research at the center is a plus for the faculty. Our university values research and it expects faculty to participate. The dynamics and/or needs of the underserved community have been research for years. The research participants have seldom benefited from the research themselves. This center gives the faculty the opportunity to be the leaders in researching the unique needs of the underserved individuals. The faculty can then utilize the research results to lead the design and implementation of interventions that meet the unique needs of the underserved. Yearly evaluation of faculty includes documentation of research experience. The center provides the faculty with the unique combination of clinical teaching and research in nursing.

LESSONS LEARNED DURING THE DEVELOPMENT OF EXPERIENCE ENGAGING THE FACULTY

Factors Discouraging Change

Being entrenched in traditional clinical nursing education within an institution, the concept of taking nursing students into a neighborhood and residents homes was unusual. Faculty members whose experience had been predominantly in the hospital setting were hesitant to go into the neighborhood. The hospital clinical experience was their comfort zone, the neighborhood an unknown area. Reaching out to the new and unlimited possibilities for nursing education in the neighborhoods of the Housing Authority of Winston-Salem was not a universal priority, and that may never change. Some faculty, however, did become more comfortable with the idea.

Factors Facilitating Change

EDUCATION

During the center's first year of operation, Dr. Mary Anne Gauthier and Dr. Margaret Ann Mahoney of Northeastern University and the Center for Community Health, Education, Research, and Service (CCHERS) presented a workshop for the faculty. The workshop "CCHERS from Boston" provided our faculty the opportunity to learn how Northeastern University had successfully taken their clinical education experiences into the neighborhood. Dr. Gauthier and Dr. Mahoney shared the ideas and experiences they had encountered. This workshop provided our faculty the opportunity to visualize how Winston-Salem State University could take the clinical education of the nursing students to the neighborhood. This was a new idea for some of our faculty members who were accustomed to the traditional clinical nursing experiences.

ORIENTATION

The faculty expressed apprehension and uncertainty when they first came to the center. To help with their acclimation, the director took them on tours, introduced them to key people, and helped them to identify residents with whom their students could initiate visits. Faculty members were able to promote continuity of care of residents and to help the students see how their interventions contributed to meeting the long-term objectives for health promotion of residents.

During the first semester, each course had one faculty member as clinical instructor for all their students who came to the center. Being at the center for the entire semester gave the faculty members time to develop their creativity and identify ways to provide meaningful clinical experiences for the students. This amount of contact also provided time for trust to start to develop between faculty, staff, and residents. Once the residents get to know you and trust you, they are more receptive and excited about participating in health promotion programs.

OWNERSHIP

The fact that the center belongs to the faculty and students of Winston-Salem State University to serve residents was stressed. The ownership of the facility and the increased degree of freedom to practice the independent aspects of the nursing role were seen as assets. Some faculty members discovered that the neighborhood had many health education treasures.

Some faculty came to value the community experiences as they saw other agencies increase their respect of the efforts. The more collaboratively the center works with community agencies, the more respect the agencies develop for the center. As the agencies discover that the staff, faculty, and students operate the center under the auspices of the university, they are developing more respect for the university as a provider of health care.

FUTURE DEVELOPMENTS

The Nurse-Managed Center for the Elderly has served as the foundation for the development of a University/Community Wellness Center. This new center integrates the Nurse-Managed Center for the Elderly and the Winston-Salem State University Student Center. It now serves as a state-of-the-art clinical practice site for students.

The future of the center lies in providing intergenerational care for all underserved groups. Since North Carolina and Winston-Salem have one of the highest infant mortality rates, it is projected that a Center for Healthy Babies will become the next major emphasis of the Wellness Center. There has also been an increase in the Hispanic community in the Winston-Salem area. The Steering Committee of the Center believes it must expand the focus to include this population.

The center will also serve as a practice site for faculty within the Division of Health Science. Research opportunities, as the university develops graduate programs, are a high priority. It is also anticipated that the center will become a practice site for other institutions offering health care programs.

Utilizing technology to connect the neighborhood and the University/ Community Wellness Center with students and faculty is a future goal. The Wellness Center will also become connected with other health care facilities to enhance the access for its clients to health care.

SUMMARY

The Nurse-Managed Center for the Elderly provides services designed to promote health, prevent disease, and maintain a healthier life style for residents in public housing. Health services offered through this neighborhood-based center consist of assessment, screening, education, counseling, basic health care, and referrals. The university's health professional faculty and students offer these services, with nurses providing the majority of services. The center provides clinical experiences and research opportunities for the nursing faculty and students as well as developing effective partnerships with community agencies. The center, subscribing to the goals in *Healthy People 2000*, provides the means to promote preventive services by improving access to primary care and removing cultural barriers to preventive care.

REFERENCES

Alfaro-LeFevre, R. (1999). *Critical Thinking in Nursing*, 2nd Ed. Philadelphia, W. B. Saunders

American Nurses Association. (1987). *Position statement on Primary Care*. Washington, DC: Author.

Lienhard School of Nursing, Pace University. (1992). *Patient Satisfaction Survey. Workbook on Establishing a Nurse Managed Center*. Pleasantville, N.J.: Briarcliff.

Luckmann, Joan (1999). *Transcultural Communication In Nursing*. Albany, NY: Delmar Publishers.

McEwen, Melanie (1998). *Community-Based Nursing: An Introduction*. Philadelphia, W. B. Saunders Company.

McKnight, J. (1995). *The Careless Society and Its Counterfeits*. New York: Harper Collins Publisher, Inc.

National League for Nursing. (1993). *A Vision for Nursing Education*. New York: Author.

U.S. Department of Health and Human Services (USDHHS). (1990). *Healthy People 2000: National Health Promotion and Disease Prevention Objectives. Summary Report*. Washington, D.C: Government Printing Office.

6

Valuing Incremental Change: The Experience of the University of Rhode Island

Jeanne M. Leffers, Marylee Evans,

Deborah Godfrey Brown, and Diane C. Martins

The University of Rhode Island possesses several unique attributes that define its strengths and abilities as well as facilitate or encumber movement towards curriculum change. A land grant institution of higher learning and the only state university, URI balances the constraints of conservative legislative funding with the expectation of service as a resource to the public and private sector of Rhode Island. Students and faculty are acutely aware of the benefits of political activism.

Working within the country's smallest state in geographic area, the College of Nursing provides service to and maintains affiliations in all counties of the state. Consequently, the regions served include rural, urban, and suburban, each with specific needs. A student, for example, might have a clinical practicum for the childbearing course in the city about 40 miles distant from the rural setting of his or her clinical practicum for mental health nursing the following day. Such diverse clinical settings prepare the students for future roles in a variety of settings.

The College of Nursing is the only state institution to offer nursing programs at the graduate level, thereby creating a strong allegiance with many nurse leaders in the state. The College of Nursing has strong collaborative relationships with many acute care institutions. URI nursing students not only readily gain employment in hospitals in the state but also are shown preference by some facilities. In order to maintain those strong ties, the College of Nursing has sought to retain placements in acute care settings while enhancing the partnership quality of community-based learning experiences.

Rhode Island lacks true Neighborhood Health Centers in the comprehensive understanding of the concept. There are a number of health centers throughout the state that are administered through the Neighborhood Health Plan managed care program. These are, however, primary care clinical settings that lack the broad preventive focus of a genuine community health center. Graduate nursing students enrolled in the family nurse practitioner program have strong partnerships with many of these primary care sites in such a way that limits the access for undergraduate student experiences.

The College of Nursing has a long history of service to vulnerable populations through faculty and graduate and undergraduate students. Some faculty serve as volunteers on Boards of Directors of many agencies. These partnerships are very important to maintain. In addition, the focus of the senior level community health course has become a practicum in the care of vulnerable populations including children, the elderly, the handicapped, the underserved, and the culturally diverse.

With consideration of the above factors, the College of Nursing changed the undergraduate curriculum while maintaining salient features of the program. The move to more community-based learning experiences for students brought about changes in traditional inpatient sites that broadened the focus to multiple community experiences. For example, home visits have become regular features of each of the institution-based clinical practicums. This allows students to view health/illness as part of the total lived experience of their clients. Students learn about the impact of health problems across generations of a family and a community as a whole. The changes had been planned prior to the participation of four key faculty members in the Northeastern University Summer Institute of July, 1996, however, the philosophy of the "Nursing in the Neighborhood" model served to sharpen our commitment to change.

THE STUDENT EXPERIENCE

The following example of one recent graduate's experience may help to illustrate how the new curriculum both develops the community focus early in the curriculum and enhances the collaborative service role of students to agency at the conclusion of the program.

Sally entered our program from the Navy where she was a medical corpsman. While she was comfortable in the health care setting, she was as apprehensive as any of the other "pioneers" in our new curriculum. In the first clinical course outside the college nursing arts laboratory setting, she selected the most urban of our clinical placements for the sophomore level health promotion course practicum. There she worked in a variety of neighborhood settings including: a Head Start Center where she taught 3- and 4-year-olds about germs and the importance of hand washing and proper use of tissues; a center for immigrants and refugees where she assisted with health screenings by taking blood pressure readings, glucometer readings, and client histories; a senior center where she met an older adult willing to participate in a health assessment and gave influenza immunizations; clinical experiences in an elementary school, a visit to an occupational health clinic at a manufacturing site; and a cardiac rehabilitation program. At the end of the first clinical, she eagerly anticipated her entry into the next course which is based in an acute care setting. Yet, she brought the perspective of health promotion, prevention, and community focus with her.

Four semesters later, Sally returned to the same community for her senior community health experience. During the intervening semesters, Sally's contacts with the community included a follow-up home visit to a patient discharged from her care in the hospital, attending a patient support group, and visiting a new mother and infant with a family outreach nurse. Her practicum in mental health nursing was spent in a community setting while her other experiences with maternity, pediatric, and medical surgical patients were primarily in acute care settings.

Sally elected to return to the urban setting for her final semester. In addition to caring for clients in the home care setting, she chose to return to the same Head Start Center she had worked in two years prior, but this time she came as a confident senior. During Sally's first experience there, her clinical instructor and the health aide on site at the center served as mentors for her. When she returned, she became an advisor to the center that provided services to 280 children each day. Her weekly activities there included some of the same activities such as health screenings of children, teaching presentations, and providing assessments for hurt or ill children. Sally was able, however, to provide a much-needed service to this aggregate setting. Her increased knowledge and experience in assessment and implementation, plus her skills developed during her pediatric clinical practicum, provided her with greater expertise to serve the agency. She, with the help of another student, compiled a comprehensive reference manual for the health aide using materials that other University of Rhode Island nursing students had provided in previous years, but in greater depth and organization. Since the health aide did not have extensive reference materials about such issues as common childhood illnesses, rationale for screenings, community resources, and information for parents, Sally's manual became the health resource of information for the staff there.

OVERVIEW OF EDUCATIONAL INSTITUTION

As noted in the introduction, the University of Rhode Island is considered a leader in public education in the state. We are one of three state institutions of higher learning that educate undergraduate nurses, but the only one to offer a BS, MS, and PhD in nursing as well as programs preparing graduates for certification as a Family Nurse Practitioner and Certified Nurse Midwife. We offer entry into clinical courses every semester, so all classes are offered every semester allowing about 100 students to graduate each year.

The campus of the University of Rhode Island is located in the more rural part of the state, however, we provide clinical experiences for students in almost all areas of the state. Thus, we have urban, suburban, and more rural clinical settings for practice. Our former traditional community health experiences have been linked to various Visiting Nurse Associations throughout Rhode Island. Prior to the restructuring patterns for the '90s, these agencies were independent nursing agencies operating geographically in more than eight regions of the state. We contracted with five agencies for many years to allow our students the opportunity to provide nursing care to individuals and families in the home setting. During the 1980s, we formalized our activities in each specific community when students worked with a group or aggregate placement in addition to a home care assignments. The development of many of these partnerships will be discussed in more detail further in this chapter. Thus, for the past two decades we have served various communities of the state by locating our five or six community clinical placements in all five counties of Rhode Island. In addition, our institutional practice sites are located in three different counties up to 40 miles from one another.

Although the University of Rhode Island is a state university program, there are a significant number of out-of-state students. Strong outreach efforts and a successful 30-year-old talent development program on campus have increased the number of ethnically diverse students. In recent years, nursing graduates include young women and men who have immigrated from Laos, Cambodia, Eritrea, Columbia, China, Guatemala, Liberia, the Dominican Republic and the former Soviet Union.

History of Change

Over the past 20 years, the undergraduate curriculum at the University of Rhode Island College of Nursing has evolved from a traditional, block-style "medical model" to a more nursing-focused, block-style model, and finally to a more community-based model. In addition to changing the course sequencing and content, the latest curriculum revision necessitated a change in faculty practice, as more faculty needed to adapt their traditional education and practice experiences to non-traditional settings.

Early in 1994, the college scheduled a meeting of faculty and representatives from a variety of clinical agencies to discuss the changing health care delivery system and its impact on the educational needs of students. Two primary issues emerged: 1) many jobs for new graduates were moving from traditional institution settings into community agencies and locales, and 2) baccalaureate graduates were expected to take on leadership roles with more managerial responsibilities. This meeting, in conjunction with a review of the National League for Nursing accreditation requirements (NLN, 1992) and the American Association of Colleges of Nursing's Essentials document (AACN, 1987), formed the basis for discussions among the undergraduate faculty concerning how to change the curriculum. The active involvement of the faculty from the very beginning of the process, along with the input from clinical agency experts, helped to facilitate the initiation of a minor curriculum change.

The fall semester of 1994 began with a continuation of the discussion at the spring meeting, specifically identification of major areas needing change. The overall behavioral outcomes for the undergraduate program were revised and updated. From this base, discussions ensued concerning potential options for change. Debate focused upon making incremental changes to the existing curriculum versus a major revision to the entire program. Faculty resistance, as always, stemmed primarily from "territorial" issues. Concerns included such questions as: Will I lose my area of interest? Will my specific expertise be needed and or valued in a new curriculum? How do we balance our educational backgrounds and practice experiences with the need for changes to meet the evolving health care delivery system? Will accrediting agencies such as the NLN permit faculty to teach outside our traditional areas of expertise? Undergraduate faculty meetings were scheduled more frequently than usual to allow time for extensive discussion and sharing of ideas and concerns. Any change had to be developed and owned by the faculty.

Overall, we agreed that some fairly major changes were necessary. More community experiences were necessary, but that did not mean that all courses had to be community-based. All faculty did not have to teach in the community. Outcomes for community-based exposure and experiences were developed for each level (sophomores, juniors, and seniors). Recognition of the uniqueness of Rhode Island and our commitment to the state as a whole community were incorporated into our planning. Also considered throughout the planning process was the need for increased leadership and managerial experiences, especially at the senior level. Finally, we agreed that more emphasis was needed on an across-the-lifespan approach in each course and at each level. Development of new courses was done sequentially, beginning with the freshman year. We reexamined the prerequisites for the nursing major, but made no significant changes. We also considered how discussions at the university level to change the general education requirements for all students might impact our program. In the fall of 1994, we developed four new courses for the freshman and sophomore years. Three involved significant revisions to existing courses while one health and physical assessment at the sophomore level was developed as the first clinical course. The content had been previously integrated into other courses across the curriculum, but students did not emerge with the whole picture or feeling that they could integrate health assessment and interviewing with a complete head-to-toe assessment. Emphasis at this level was the identification of normal patterns across the lifespan.

Faculty representatives met with consultants from Northeastern University to learn more about the "Nursing in the Neighborhood" model. Although many aspects of their program were impossible to emulate in Rhode Island, the philosophical underpinnings mirrored our own. In the spring of 1995, the upper division courses were developed. While faculty still voiced some concerns about restructuring and specific course changes, unanimous approval was given for the new curriculum. Again, though resistance was encountered and dealt with throughout the process, faculty recognized the need for change, and adequate time for discussion was allowed and encouraged even when we had to revisit several concerns again.

During this time frame, we were also seeking student input concerning the existing curriculum and where or how they would like to see changes made. In addition to the usual course and overall program evaluation tools, we actively sought student participation on the college's Curriculum Committee and Program Evaluation Committee. Informal feedback was also received through other committees and organizations such as the Student Affairs Committee and the Student Nurse's Association. Their major concerns centered on the development of clinical skills and appropriate preparation for the job market.

Students currently in the program at that time were not initially asked to change to a new curriculum and did not express concern about the change in content for the new courses. Student resistance became more apparent as the new curriculum was implemented. Although the changes were in the catalog for new incoming students, we did find that there were students already enrolled in the college (primarily transfer students, returning or second-degree students, and students within the university) that had changed majors and were caught in the transition to the new curriculum. In the spring of 1996, the new health assessment course was taught concurrently with the former sophomore level courses. Selection by the college's Scholastic Standing Committee in the new rather than the old curriculum was based, as always, on the overall grade point average (GPA), but also upon the number of semesters the student carried a nursing code. The large number of students ready to enter the clinical courses that semester prompted this decision.

New Curriculum

Our nursing curriculum is based upon the belief that nursing is a creative activity that provides human services for the promotion of health, prevention of illness, and care of the ill. We use a systems theory framework as a conceptual base to nursing. This conceptual approach incorporates the whole person and his or her environment into the nursing process. As we prepare our students for the 21st Century, we have sought to enhance student education for increased technology, increased diversity, and greater skills for critical thinking and decision-making. As a public institution of learning, our goals include the need to serve our state by serving both the private and the public sector. We encourage collaborative working relationships with community partners. In addition, the College of Nursing faculty and students are involved in a number of interdisciplinary partnerships without the university.

Our new curriculum features an early introduction to community health with the expansion of our health promotion course, continued community experiences throughout the program, and an enhanced community health experience in the final semester. For many students, one-third to almost one-half of their clinical practicum experience may be spent in community settings. An example of the new eight semester curriculum is presented in Table 6-1.

How does clinical integrate with theory?

Each clinical course is taught concurrently with a theoretical course of the same focus. In keeping with our educational philosophy, during the first three semesters of the curriculum, students are socialized to regard health and health promotion activities as a primary focus of nursing care. This sets a framework of reference for all subsequent clinical courses. Senior level courses explore leadership and management theories, provide preceptor learning experiences with nurse leaders, and emphasize critical thinking and decision-making skills that the graduate must employ in future professional roles. Many of the courses retain a traditional rather than integrated model (childbearing, psychiatric mental health, medical

TABLE 6-1 University of Rhode Island College of Nursing Undergraduate Curriculum

First Year

Semester 1
  Human Anatomy (4)
  General Sociology (3)
  Introductory Chemistry (3)

  Freshman Seminar (1)

  General Education Elective (3)

Semester 2
  Human Physiology (3)
  Human Physiology Laboratory (1)
  Introduction to Organic
    Chemistry (3)
  General Psychology (3)
  Nursing 103: Professional
    Practice in Health and Illness (3)
  General Education Elective (3)

Second Year

Semester 1
  Introductory Medical
    Microbiology (4)
  Statistics (3)

  Nur 203: Comprehensive
  Health Assessment (3)
  General Nutrition (3)

  Developmental Psychology (3)

Semester 2
  Nur 213: Pathophysiology (3)

  Nur 223: Health Promotion
    Nursing:
  Strategies and Interventions (3)
  Nur 224: Practicum in Health
    Promotion Nursing (3)
  Nur 273: Critical Thinking and
    Research in Nursing (3)
  General Education Course (3)

Third Year

Semester 1
  Nur 323: Health Restoration:
  Health Nursing Strategies and I
    interventions (6)
  Nur 324: Practicum in Health
    Restoration
  Nursing (6)
  Pharmacology and
    Therapeutics (2)
  Free Elective (3)

Semester 2
  Nur 333 Psychiatric Mental
    Nursing (3)

  Nur 334: Practicum in Psychiatric
    Mental Health Nursing (3)
  Nur 343: Nursing in Childbearing
    and Reproductive Health (3)

  Nur 344: Practicum in
    Childbearing and Reproductive
    Health Nursing (3)
  Pharmacology & Therapeutics
    II (2)
  Free Elective (3)

(continued)

TABLE 6-1 *(continued)*

Fourth Year	
Semester 1	*Semester 2*
Nur 423: Chronic Health Alterations: Strategies and Interventions (3)	Nur 443: Nursing of Vulnerable Populations in the Home and the Community (3)
Nur 424: Practicum in Nursing of Older Adults with Health Alterations (3)	Nur 444: Praticum in Nursing of Vulnerable Populations (3)
Nur 434: Practicum in Nursing of Children with Health Alterations (3)	Nur 454: Theories, Issues, and Practice in Professional Nursing (3)
2 General Education Courses (6)	2 General Education courses (6)

A total of 125 credits is required for graduation. All credit hours are noted in parentheses. The 60 credits in nursing listed above are required in the sequence given. Also offered in the College of Nursing are elective courses in Human Sexuality, Aging and Health, and Impact of Death on Behavior as well as a Directed Independent Study.

surgical, and pediatric practicums), however, the themes of health promotion and home and community care are integrated throughout the seven semesters of nursing courses.

Curriculum changes

Although students in the former curriculum began their nursing study with a nursing concepts course (Nursing 103), the new course introduces concepts such as communication, teaching-learning strategies, critical thinking, the health system, and community-focused approaches. Next, the students complete a comprehensive health assessment course in the nursing arts laboratory setting. During their third semester of nursing courses (fourth semester of the program), they enroll in the new health promotion course (Nursing 223) and clinical practicum (Nursing 224). This practicum provides students with the opportunity to practice communication, assessment, and teaching learning strategies learned in the prior courses in addition to the concepts taught in the concurrent health promotion theory course.

Prior to much of the health care reform of the '90s and the move to community-based nursing, our college already had in place a health promotion theory course and practicum taught at the sophomore level for the past 10 years. For most of those 10 years, a three-credit Health Promotion theory course was aligned with a three-credit health Promotion practicum to give students knowledge and practice in the areas of health promotion and prevention to clients of all ages. The main emphasis was on wellness and primary and secondary levels of prevention. Nursing students engaged in formal and informal health teaching and counseling and performed a variety of screenings. The unit of service was the individual client across the life span within the context of families, aggregates, and communities. The practicum setting was community-based rather than in any institution. The community experience, however, was an eclectic one in which the placements were not necessarily limited to one community but occurred wherever a placement was found to meet the objectives of the course.

During the same semester, a fundamentals of nursing course was taught providing students with two credits of beginning knowledge of nursing practice and a one-credit clinical for the development and practice of basic patient care skills. This course focused primarily on traditional fundamentals content with an emphasis on nursing process and beginning assessment skills. The practicum focused mainly on the development of psychomotor skills in the on-campus nursing arts laboratory followed by a few weeks in a nursing home caring for one individual patient for the entire rotation. This gave students the opportunity to directly apply the skills learned in the lab as well a practice therapeutic communication and use the self as the major therapeutic tool with their patients. This four- to five-week rotation also allowed the students to experience and analyze the helping relationship through all phases including termination. The nursing process was also applied throughout the rotation so students could work through all phases from assessment to evaluation. Because students provided care to only one individual, a nursing care plan could be developed, implemented, evaluated, revised, and shared with the nursing staff. Students were able to see the impact of their care and the positive changes in their patients.

The curriculum framework used for structuring this sequence of nursing courses within the nursing major was systems theory. This theory dictated that the unit of service and study for the freshman and sophomore years was client and client-nurse. This preceded subsequent courses that focused on the more complex family and community components. There was also no theoretical framework unifying the courses together in theory. Indeed, they ran as separate entities, complete unto themselves.

Before our curriculum change, a minor change was made that reduced the health promotion practicum to only one credit. Further complicating the educational focus, both the one-credit fundamentals and one-credit health promotion courses were to be offered on the same day. One clinical instructor had the same students for both courses. Cost containment efforts to better utilize faculty was the impetus for this arrangement. As might be expected, this was educationally unsound and unwieldy to manage, providing more impetus for curriculum change.

In the new curriculum, the fundamentals course was dissolved, moving the content to the Nursing 103 and health assessment courses and deferring the "hands-on" patient care skills to the junior year. The health promotion theory course continued at the sophomore level and remained somewhat intact while the practicum returned to its former three-credit status.

The health promotion courses were expanded to include an overall introduction to community-based nursing practice. Since this is the philosophy of care adopted by the faculty for its undergraduate curriculum, the basic premises of this philosophy are spelled out in this course and applied in its health promotion practicum. The course content includes principles of community-based care such as self-care, levels of prevention, continuity of care from an interdisciplinary team, and community support networks. This serves as a foundation upon which the rest of the curriculum is built. Students learn to use tools such as family assessments and community assessments. This community framework socializes the student in the first clinical course to look beyond the individual level, recognize the importance of prevention, and view health as a focus of nursing.

An emphasis in Health Promotion was also no longer primarily centered around the individual as the unit of service but around family and community units of service as well. To directly apply this theory to practice, the students must do detailed assignments focused on the individual (health promotion assessment), family (family assessment at a home visit), and community (assessment as a group project). Each assessment culminates in identification of risk factors, nursing diagnoses, client outcomes, and interventions for primary, secondary and/or tertiary prevention.

Clinical practice is no longer eclectic but is restricted to one smaller geographic area or "neighborhood" for all clinical placements. The word "neighborhood" varies from once clinical group to the next. Some "neighborhoods" are large rural areas encompassing more that one town but all sharing one set of resources. Others are smaller urban areas where the resources are closer together. As a state, Rhode Island is so small that most of it can be utilized (whether rural or urban) in one clinical course.

Educational Strengths of New Curriculum

One of the strengths of this new curriculum is that students come to the first clinical practicum with skills in teaching and learning, communication, group dynamics, and physical assessment. During the semester prior to the Health Promotion Courses, students take a comprehensive three-credit (2-hour theory, 3-hour lab) health assessment course. This course introduces them to systematic history-taking and the skills to perform a complete, head-to-toe assessment across the lifespan. This provides good preparation to begin working with clients in the community and effectively implement prevention strategies across all three levels.

Intervening Semesters between Community-Based Education

During the three semesters between the health promotion experience and the senior community health course, students complete medical surgical, psychiatric mental health, pediatric, and maternity courses. During each of these semesters, students make a home visit and participate in some community experience. In each of the medical surgical experiences, the students make a visit to a client they have cared for in the hospital to identify the effectiveness of their patient teaching and to identify needs specific to the home setting. They also attend a support group meeting pertinent to the adult population. The students in the senior level medical surgical course begin their clinical experience in a sub-acute setting to better understand the long-term needs of clients. Most of the clinical experiences in the mental health practicum are community- and home-based. All students attend an Alcoholics Anonymous meeting and visit a community agency such as a rape crisis center or women's resource center as well. The students in the childbearing and reproductive health practicum make a home care visit to a postpartum family, visit childbirth education classes, and visit an ambulatory service for women's health such as prenatal clinics, midwifery practices, and diagnostic centers.

New Senior Level Courses

Prior to the curriculum change, our community health faculty were able to provide our students with a sound clinical practicum in community health nursing. The course was taught, however, during the seventh semester concurrently with their maternity course and prior to their pediatric experience and long-term care experiences in the eight semester. We found that students assigned their community course less importance and failed to achieve the most from this experience. Not only have we returned the community health course to the final semester but we have also increased expectations of student performance. In our new curriculum, students often provide care for patients in the home care setting with more complex problems demanding greater skill levels. The new clinical practicum includes a variety of focused written assignments that sharpen their thinking about family, social, environmental, and health policy issues. Increased focus is placed upon the empowerment of clients using the philosophy of Paulo Freire (1970).

Each student is assigned a home care patient from his or her respective agency. With our focus upon vulnerable populations, the home care patient they select has complex biophysical and psychosocial needs. The student makes a home visit each week usually at the beginning of the clinical day. In addition, each student selects an aggregate setting in the same community to work in for the semester. In this setting, the student identifies in collaboration with the clients and staff of the agency a community health-planning project (Godfrey-Brown et al., 1997). During this semester, students employ strategies to encourage empowerment of the clients they are serving.

An Example of Practicum Development

Kathy commuted to Rhode Island from nearby Connecticut for her education. She elected to follow a patient requiring extensive wound care treatment for infection and complications following colon resection for carcinoma. In this family setting, she not only provided complex interventions for his wound care, colostomy, and MRSA infection but also identified issues related to the demands upon the family, his emotional and social needs, and community resources. She usually visited him from 8:00 A.M. to 9:00 A.M. each week. Kathy then traveled to the aggregate, in her "community" from two years prior. The aggregate she selected to work with was a school for severely handicapped children whose nursing needs included assessments, medication administration, gastric feedings, nasopharyngeal suctioning, and, in some cases, ventilator care. Kathy assisted the nursing staff in direct patient care, however, her focus was upon the children as a population group. Taking note of the fact that many of the children were allergic to latex and that their environment was filled with latex products, she consulted with the staff of the agency to identify how she might intervene as an advocate for these children. Throughout the semester, she researched the topic, collaborated with the interdisciplinary team at the school, and prepared a comprehensive presentation for the entire school staff about the risks of latex allergy for students and nursing staff. She then obtained a film for viewing; created displays of medical products commonly used by students that contain latex and another display showing their latex-free substitutes; assembled a resource binder containing NIOSH and OSHA policies about latex, research articles, and fact sheets; and provided the school with a subscription to a periodical about latex allergy. Her five hours at the agency each week not only provided her the opportunity to work with a vulnerable population, assess, plan and implement interventions but also to assist the staff in changing school policy.

Concurrent Senior Level Courses

Concurrently with the senior level community health course, students complete a combined theory and practicum leadership course. Each student selects an area of interest in nursing. Faculty then matches the student with a nurse leader preceptor in that area. Students spend four hours weekly identifying leadership and management skills that they will employ as professional nurses. Many of the nurse managers that students elect to work with are in community-based settings while some are in acute care settings. Both this experience and the selection of an aggregate that the student makes in the community health setting allow the student to focus his or her learning and gain experience in his or her own interest area.

For example, one student, Mike, sought a career in pediatric nursing. For his community experience, he elected to have his home care experience in the pediatric home care services and work at a Head Start Center for his aggregate. For the leadership course, he worked with a nurse manager of the pediatric intensive care unit at the hospital where he spent his practicum in pediatric nursing. In addition, he developed an independent study to learn more about pediatric oncology and worked with a nurse specialist in that area. Thus, he was able to use his final semester to increase his expertise in the area of nursing he planned to pursue.

What Is a Neighborhood Assignment in Our Program?

As noted previously, we place our students in all counties of the state. Our urban partnerships differ from the experiences of those students in the more suburban and rural settings. We have a long history of collaboration with many of these agencies and did not sever ties after we established our new curriculum. Thus, a challenge has been to enhance a community model while continuing many prior relationships. In some areas, we have strengthened our collaboration significantly while, in others, we are still developing better models. An example of a strengthened relationship may serve to better explain this.

In Providence, our capital city and most urban clinical placement area, we have partnered with the Genesis Center for about 14 years. This center is a multi-service family-based center where immigrants and refugees learn English and job training skills. Our involvement with the center began not long after its founding in 1982. The original contact with the Genesis Center occurred when two Providence VNA nurses provided non-traditional VNA outreach in the community of Providence. The nurses created a clinic at the Office of Refugee Resettlement to service the large influx of refugees from Southeast Asia. This clinic initially served as an outreach clinic run by the VNA nurses in addition to those in senior centers and high-rise apartment buildings for blood pressure screening and follow-up. They soon realized, however, that the refugees were struggling with many complex issues such as adaptation to a new and vastly different culture, problems with immigration regulations, differences in health and illness practices, and misunderstanding of cultural practices of their new environment. Frequently, the new arrivals were being contacted by social service for reports of neglect of their children for reasons such as going barefoot in the winter and leaving their young children to supervise babies. Noting the needs of the new immigrants, these nurses received grant money to fund growth of their clinic. They asked nursing students and URI faculty to not only help in the clinic but also to serve as advocates for the immigrants by educating health professionals about cultural misunderstandings between them and the health care providers in Rhode Island. The URI students and the nurses co-sponsored a statewide conference for all health professionals at the university called "East meets West." When the grant money ended and the clinic was closed, faculty and nursing students continued to serve at the center. We now have students from a variety of courses serving there. During their health promotion course, they assist with health screenings and spend time in the day care center. During their senior level community health course, several spend the semester developing community health planning projects. Students in the intervening courses return to assist with health fairs, ongoing research projects, and peer health educator training. Senior students are involved with advocacy for immigrants and refugees, participation with a state Department of Health Minority Health grant, health policy formation for the agency, health education, and consultation with individual clients. Most of the students electing placement at the center are immigrants themselves. In particular, two students are the children of Genesis School graduates. By returning to the center as college seniors, they model to the newly arrived clients both the value of their parent's efforts and hope for the future. Presently, a URI nursing faculty member volunteers there to provide consultation, referral, and follow-up services. Faculty and graduate student assistants to better understand cultural needs related to health are conducting a funded research project there. The center recognized the nursing faculty member with their fifth Genesis Award for outstanding service.

PARTNERSHIPS

Throughout the state, the College of Nursing has ongoing partnerships with a variety of agencies and programs. Of the five municipalities with the highest rates of childhood poverty, nursing students serve all but the one too distant from campus (Kid's Count Data Book, 1998). In addition, two areas of the state are quite inclusive, one located on an island, the other a rural area near the coastal beaches. Residents of these areas tend to utilize services specific to their own "neighborhood," creating opportunities for nursing students to use these areas as their neighborhood model.

Headstart Programs

Nursing faculty members created the partnerships with various Headstart Program in the late 1970s to create a non-traditional placement for the community health nursing students for their aggregate and home care experiences. In the Providence program, the Headstart staff quickly found many activities that would benefit the children, the parents, or the staff. This included teaching health issues in the classroom or parents meetings, writing newsletters, health aid inservices, or screening for health problems. Every semester, the social service staff would suggest needy families that each of the eight students would visit in their homes. Sometimes the need would be physical (i.e., asthma) with a child with high absenteeism or, at times, a family would be selected because the staff wanted the parents to have an opportunity to see role modeling for parenting, (nutrition, hygiene, shopping, budgeting, homework). Home visits were also suggested for children with neglect issues or for families with untreated infectious disease. Nursing students continued home visits for one semester to that family addressing multiple issues. One example is when a nursing student originally visited a home due to recurrent pediculosis infestation. After her assessment, she realized that the family needed assistance with shampooing, washing of all laundry, and spraying the rugs and stuffed animals as well as education on prevention of future infestations. This student also identified nutrition needs that included insufficient knowledge of good nutrition, creating and following an affordable food budget, and locating affordable healthy foods. A member of the nursing faculty serves on the Health Advisory Committee for the Providence Headstart Program to plan and enforce health policies, writing health program objectives and making recommendations at the administrative level for the health of the children.

With this almost 20-year relationship with the Headstart Program, we sought to further collaborate in our new curriculum. Now we have students from both the health promotion course and the senior community health course at the center. Sally's experience is an example of our involvement there. Similar examples occur at the Headstart programs that we partner with in four other communities. Our long-term ongoing relationship with these partners works well not only as an educational opportunity for our students but also to better serve the vulnerable populations of Rhode Island.

Partnerships with a School System

A partnership with an urban school department began in the early 1980s to provide school health experiences for the community health nursing students. The student nurses originally worked solely in the health office but soon began to extend to health education classes, teen parent groups, pregnant teen groups, and parent education presentations. Presently, we have student placements in elementary, middle, and high schools throughout the state. Sophomore students spend a day with a school nurse in order to learn about the health risks for school age children and adolescents. As seniors, some students elect to return to a school setting for their aggregate experience. Students have planned and assisted with immunization clinics, written grants to decrease gang enrollment by developing an after school activity program for students, and designed and advocated for a comprehensive nutrition program in a middle school that will change the snacks available in vending machines, alter food choices served in lunch program, and increase the nutrition education program in home economics classes. Others have taught classes, established school wide health newsletters, and created resource manuals for teachers.

Partnerships with the Homeless: Shelters, Soup Kitchens, and Traveler's Aid

More than a decade ago, a nursing faculty member began collaboration with the Travelers Aid Society of Rhode Island to determine health needs of the homeless in Rhode Island. Initially a service and research interest, the partnership increased to include nursing students in their practicum experience. The faculty member served on their medical advisory committee and volunteered as a nurse on their medical outreach van, prompting the agency to allow student nurses to be involved with the van, runaway youth program, free medical clinic, dental clinic, and psychiatric clinic. The students have also assisted the agency as a whole by updating the state-wide resource manual and by coordinating health programs. A strong collaborative relationship continues. Recently, the agency hired a former university nursing student as coordinator of the health clinic. The health director of the agency and the URI faculty member have jointly presented at professional conferences about outreach services and empowerment of the homeless. The agency promotes nursing research on health experiences of homeless adults and experiences of runaway youths. This particular faculty member is on the Board of Directors of the Rhode Island Coalition for the Homeless.

Soup Kitchens

Originally, the student nurses volunteered in the soup kitchens to help with meal preparation, serving, and clean up, but gradually the soup kitchen staff began to request screening for the clients. Eventually, the soup kitchens asked for programs for their workers to help with OSHA regulations for food servers and to improve their communications with difficult clients. Faculty and students volunteered at a clinic at a shelter for the homeless, and an RN student from URI remained there while in school and after her graduation.

Currently, we have students serving in shelters in four areas of the state. The students frequently sponsor food and clothing drives on campus to support the programs at these sites. The faculty of the College of Nursing strongly encourages such community service initiatives by our students.

Housing Units

Student nurses first provided outreach services to the senior adult, low income, and disabled residents in high-rise apartment and other public housing units in cooperation with visiting nurses. Students made home visits to home-bound clients and assisted visiting nurses with health screenings and referrals. The university health promotion partnership provides services to residents of these apartments in their exercise program for older adults. Undergraduate students work cooperatively with this program for community placements. In our new curriculum, a student helped to evaluate the strategies used by the partnership team in recruitment and retention of participants.

Visiting Nurse Agencies

The Visiting Nurse agencies in the state have a long history of collaboration with the College of Nursing faculty and students. Many of the staff at these agencies are graduates of the university, encouraging continued collaboration. Community health faculty members at URI continue to serve on the Board of Directors of most of the Visiting Nurse agencies. The recent proliferation of private or joint venture home care agencies has increased the need for mutual support between the college of nursing and the visiting nurse associations.

These are only some examples of the partnerships we have created and maintained over the years. We currently serve six communities through our student practicums. In each of these communities we have students serving in six to eight agencies so that we reach out to about 45 or more aggregate settings each semester. We have found that partnerships are maintained and grow when the faculty realize and support the community's recognition of their own needs. The sustained relationship is nurtured best when the faculty commits to the agency/community at a level that goes beyond solely creating a placement for the nursing student for the semester. The populations we serve benefit from a caring, ongoing, committed relationship between academia and the community we serve. Partnerships allow for a faculty member's expertise to be shared with the community and allow for the agency strengths and expertise to be shared with the faculty and student.

EVALUATION OF CHANGES

Now that we have followed our first class through to graduation, we have been able to begin to evaluate the new program. Since we have had a strong commitment to community settings throughout the state, we did not have to work hard to create new community partners. We simply changed some student learning roles and sought new learning opportunities through existing (and some new) partnerships. To evaluate these changes, we have examined the results upon our students, our faculty, and the agencies and communities we serve.

Impact upon Students

Student performance is evaluated at the end of each course according to course specific objectives related to the seven outcomes used in the college of nursing: professional role and leadership; theoretical knowledge; nursing process; intra-inter personal relationships; societal responsibility; research; and professional responsibility. Within these objectives criteria related to critical thinking, communication skills, and therapeutic skill development are evaluated. Further, faculty conduct ongoing evaluation of student performance as a whole throughout the implementation of the new curriculum. We address criteria previously mentioned as well as their increased adoption of a health promotion and prevention philosophy, community knowledge, and recognition of the health/illness continuum rather than a pathophysiology model of care.

Advantages noted thus far include better student communication and assessment skills at the beginning of the acute care experiences, increased assertiveness and independence, and, by the completion of the program, a solid integration of community concepts into their nursing philosophy. They have begun their socialization into a population-based, prevention focus upon health early in their study, allowing them to incorporate this philosophy into all phases of nursing. Students have increased exposure to culturally diverse populations earlier in their experiences with healthy individuals, promoting more effective care of the patient from a different culture in the acute care setting. Our new curriculum encourages community service as a part of their nursing role.

Certain disadvantages, however, need to be improved as we continue to modify our changes. Students, in their eagerness to take on the assumed roles they see reflected in the media (such as the popular television show "ER"), cannot wait for their hospital experience. Until students identify themselves as "nurse" we see that they lack the investment in their education. An example is one student in our health promotion course who, upon completing a physical assessment of a gentleman at the adult day care center, exclaimed, "I touched my first foot." She failed to see herself in the nursing role until she had experienced direct care. Since we are currently seeing the first of our new students complete the program, we are beginning to identify strengths and weaknesses. Obvious strengths have been noted above. We are pleased to see our students expand their role in the community and believe that they will be better prepared as professional nurses. A weakness is our ability to change the outlook of students and faculty who define "real" nursing as that which takes place only in acute care settings. Both students and faculty need to reorient thinking to see the importance of assessment and interventions in all settings.

All students are required to take the same clinical courses, however, as noted above, the settings vary from urban to rural. These differences in settings account for the differences in students' experiences. University policies allow students to register for any course section depending upon their eligibility. Consequently, students select clinical practicums by location, day and time, and clinical instructor. This means that some choose not to return to the same location. As faculty, we highly encourage the students to remain with the same community and are seeking ways to require this. For example, students may have their introductory experience in Providence (urban, inner city) at the sophomore level and elect to go to South County (rural) for their senior community experience. Their community experiences in the intervening courses may occur in any area of the state. Student responsibilities change over time, however, and some who have lived on campus move to their home or an apartment and prefer a clinical placement that does not require them to travel for up to an hour or more. So, we anticipate that, for a while, it will be the College of Nursing presence and consistency of faculty rather than the continuity of all students. Thus far, several students elected to return to their original community and, as we enter the second running of our final senior experience, more than 80% of the students elected to return to Providence for their clinical experience.

A weakness of this current curriculum has to do with the fact that students do not have an opportunity to provide physical patient care, in uniform, to someone other than a well client. Having this basic care experience delayed until the junior year and placed in an intensive six-credit medical surgical nursing practicum frustrates the students who want to become a nurse and do the "hands-on type of nursing" to fulfill the stereotype about which they have always dreamed. The junior level medical surgical nursing course also covers so much in one semester that the students are not able to absorb and assimilate the experience in such a short time. This makes the jump to acute care too big and too scary for students. Transfer of knowledge from health promotion to medical surgical practicums is also lost since students are too focused on themselves and their acute care environment and initiating any tertiary prevention strategies does not happen.

Benner (1984) explains that nurses are better able to integrate knowledge as they move from the novice level of practice to more advanced levels. Our students may be unable to integrate the vast amount of conceptual knowledge taught prior to their junior year without addressing their need for increased practice in the sophomore year. The previously mentioned student who exclaimed that she had touched her first foot was really noting the importance of physical touch in the nursing role. One of the distinctive features of nursing is the intimacy involved in the provision of care. Until our students cross that boundary, they express fear and concern about their role.

Impact upon faculty

We still have some faculty members who measure student learning by skill level and are hesitant to fully commit to the community focus. Many faculty that teach in the institutional settings are reluctant to relinquish clinical experiences traditionally considered important. All faculty involved in our new curriculum, however, agree that our students demonstrate much stronger assessment and communication skills. Our experience reflects that student outcomes meet our goals for the new curriculum.

One difficulty we experience is the continuity of faculty. Our faculty assignments are made based upon the clinical expertise that limits conti-

nuity of faculty. In recent years, the College of Nursing experienced considerable reduction in tenure track and continuing full-time faculty positions resulting in a large number of part-time clinical faculty teaching per
course. As a result, most clinical practicums may have only one or two full
time faculty and three or more part time faculty. The exceptions to this are
the first two clinical courses—our practicum in health promotion and our
first hospital-based course, health restoration. In each of these courses we
have full-time faculty in all sections. The faculty in our beginning community-based course, may not all have clinical background in community
health nursing. This limits our ability to orient our faculty to the important concepts of community health that frame our new curriculum.

This can be an advantage, however, as faculty become more socialized
to the importance of our health-focused philosophy. The changes in our
curriculum reflect those encouraged by national nursing and health care
leadership. This can serve to refocus nursing education for the future.

Impact upon the Communities We Serve

As noted previously, Rhode Island is a small state resulting in limited
human resources. Prior to the implementation of the new curriculum,
the College of Nursing already linked students to community aggregates throughout the state. Now, we have students at all levels of the
curriculum competing for placements in various settings. Further,
another nursing program has recently begun to emulate our model of
aggregate placements, increasing the numbers of students in agency settings. The potentially marvelous result of this is that nurses can and do
make a difference in the lives of people in Rhode Island. Until we create better organization in our outreach efforts, however, we are likely to
saturate the service providers who give generously of their time to teach
our students.

There is little doubt that the community health planning projects
undertaken by our senior students provide tangible reminders of the
service we provide. In order to maintain such quality service, our faculty devote a great deal of time and effort to the continuation of the partnerships.

FUTURE PLANS

The next logical step will be to define and strengthen more partnerships
throughout the state. As students become more responsible to their specific communities, the College of Nursing will be better able to increase

our service to them. We need to further develop the longitudinal commitment for individual students so that they recognize and value the community experiences that occur between the Health Promotion course (4th semester) and the Nursing of Vulnerable Populations course (8th semester) course. Institutional settings both excite and engage students in ways that often course community experiences to appear less important to beginning student nurses. Our goal is to improve our ability to prepare students for both preventive and restorative care together.

In particular, we are looking for ways to improve the transition to the acute care setting. If we can expand the health promotion course, we hope to offer a second clinical practicum day that would allow us to incorporate the tertiary level of prevention in a rehabilitation setting. In this way, the students will become more comfortable in dealing with clients who require "hands-on" care, allowing them to touch a person as patient prior to the junior year. This might reduce their fear of the acute care setting in the health restoration course. In addition, it would also link the community and acute care settings in a way that students are more likely to recognize and less likely to divide the experiences into community and "real" nursing.

Further, the College of Nursing has recently established the URI Center for Nurse Midwifery and plans to create other faculty practice settings. With the establishment of nursing centers, our students will have comprehensive community-based sites. In addition, we are seeking more collaboration with the community health clinics as the number of clients enrolled in the state program for the uninsured, RIte Care, expands. This may also create stronger neighborhood models.

We hope to increase the community service commitment of our students. Presently, the college of nursing has two community service initiatives that have been funded by the Feinstein Service Learning program on campus. One is at the Genesis Center described previously, and the other is a teen parent mentoring program in another urban area of the state. A number of students participate in these programs during the semesters between their community experiences. This service increases their collaborative role with community members, increases their commitment to a community aggregate, and extends the college of nursing outreach into vulnerable and underserved populations.

We are committed to continue our community-based approach to nursing education. In order to prepare nurse leaders for the 21st Century, we must educate students to promote health wherever people work and live. As our health care delivery system rapidly changes, the University of Rhode Island seeks to prepare our graduates for professional roles in varied settings. As the only institution in the state that prepares nurses at baccalaureate, masters, and doctoral levels, our service to the state is vital to students and citizens alike.

SUMMARY

Each school must consider curriculum change in a manner that builds on current strengths and enhances not only the learning experiences of students but also the services provided through neighborhood partnerships. The College of Nursing at the University of Rhode Island has, through an incremental change process, found ways to more effectively teach students about human diversity and health care systems and prepare them to provide health promotion, risk reduction, and disease prevention programs while also collaborating with patients in illness and disease management. As with all educational endeavors, ongoing analysis and evaluation will continue to impel forward further creativeness in curriculum change.

REFERENCES

American Association of College of Nursing (1987). *Essentials of college and university education for professional nursing: Final Report*. Washington, DC. Author.

Benner, P. (1984). *From Novice to Expert: Excellence and Power in Clinical Nursing Practice*. Menlo Park, CA: Addison-Wesley.

Freire, P. (1970). *Pedagogy of the Oppressed*. New York: Continuum.

Godfrey-Brown, Deb, Burbank, P., & Morgan, B. (1997) *Community health planning and evaluation*. pp. 117–134 in Janice M. Swanson and Mary Nies, eds. *Community Health Nursing: Promoting the Health of Aggregates*. Philadelphia: Saunders.

Kids Count Fact Book. (1998) Providence, RI: Annie Casey Foundation.

Matteson, P. (Ed.). (1995) *Teaching Nursing in the Neighborhood: the Northeastern University Model*. New York: Springer.

National League for Nursing (1992). *An agenda for nursing education reform*. New York: Author.

7

Serendipity and Courage: The Experience of American International College (Massachusatts)

Marilyn Breuer, Karen Rousseau, and Ayesha Ali

During the academic year 1995–1996, the Curriculum and Evaluation Committee of the Division of Nursing at American International College began to have serious discussion and debate about the increasing movement of nursing into the community. Although there was a wide range of opinions among faculty about how we might address that in our curriculum, we generally agreed about two broad areas. First, we would begin to explore community opportunities in the context of our curriculum and clinical experiences. Second, we understood the importance of increasing cultural awareness in the delivery of nursing into our program. The college is nestled in a predominately black community, our city has a growing multi-ethnic population, and many of our students come from diverse backgrounds.

Some of us were familiar with the Northeastern University model and, as we learned more about it, we imagined how we could integrate the model into our curriculum and into our community. We had questions, however. Did we have a sufficient number of faculty? Could we find community partners? Would there be a negative impact on students having less acute care experience? What of the value of skills learned in the community as compared with acute care? How would students move through the community and what types of experiences would be valuable? Would we have to use more adjunct faculty members? Could students be independent earlier in our curriculum sequence?

Finally, it came down to two attributes that we nourished in each other: courage and serendipity. Courage was the necessary ingredient that enabled us to move forward with an innovative curriculum in spite of our own trepidation as well as that of students and skeptical colleagues. We had to take that leap as a faculty and rely on each other's strengths, and the student's ability to take on a challenge.

Serendipity is the unexpected occurrence that provides unforeseen opportunities and challenges and is vital to our experience of teaching nursing in the neighborhood both for faculty and students. It was a serendipitous encounter in a hospital corridor between a faculty member and a hospital nursing administrator which began the collaboration between the Cultural Awareness Committee of Baystate Medical Center (BMC) and our neighborhood nursing faculty. The committee was eager to involve nursing students in its outreach to the greater community in a cultural context and to have students share in gathering information about health care issues in various cultural groups in the Springfield area.

One of our earliest experiences was in the Vietnamese community in the Forest Park area of Springfield. This is a large community of Southeast Asians, mainly Vietnamese, with a well-established Vietnamese Cultural Center that gives aide to new immigrants and helps maintain cultural ties and customs. It was serendipitous that our first group of students came to the center a few weeks before Tet, the Vietnamese New Year's celebration. The community was very involved in preparation for this day-long event which would bring Vietnamese people from all over New England for a traditional celebration. The students were invited to help in the preparations. That certainly did not fit into the student's goal of providing health care, but it did more than fit into our goal of getting to know the people and their culture. In fact, we had no more expectations for that first semester in this community than having members feel comfortable with the faculty and students and recognize that we would provide a continuing presence.

The students helped make decorations and, while involved in that activity with community members, they established a comfort level and learned about the culture. At the Tet celebration the students teamed with the Cultural Awareness Committee from BMC in taking blood pressures and disseminating health information. Students began to participate in the monthly Health Resource Day provided for the elders of the community by taking blood pressures and getting to know the elders. Two major objectives for each clinical group were to identify a teaching need and to identify community health care resources. These activities led them to another serendipitous encounter with the Southwest Neighborhood Health Center and the infectious disease nurse from the Springfield Department of Health and Human Services just as a high incidence of Hepatitis C was identified in this community. The students were able to learn how a public health problem such as this is addressed at the local level. Students were guests at the first information sessions. Students and faculty were invited to participate in the initial screening and immunization endeavors, and the students were invited by the community elders to give a presentation on Hepatitis C to the community.

That first semester brought more enriching experiences for our students than faculty ever expected. The first few weeks took courage from the students who felt insecure without the amount of structure and direction they were used to in a traditional health care setting to work with clients and families in an unfamiliar cultural environment. It also took courage from the faculty who were feeling the students' distress and wondering if learning objectives would be met. It was that openness to the serendipitous occurrences and the ability to embrace those opportunities, however, which made both students and faculty aware of the extensive possibilities to provide health care and make nursing in the neighborhood challenging, unique and rewarding to both students and faculty.

OUR MODEL OF NEIGHBORHOOD-BASED CLINICAL EDUCATION

Philosophical Tenets of Clinical Education

There are three important tenets which underline our philosophy of neighborhood-based clinical education. First is commitment to the three neighborhoods we serve and the selected group within each neighborhood: African American, Hispanic, and Vietnamese. Faculty learned from discussions in the BMC Cultural Awareness Committee and from talking to community leaders that minority community members are very distrustful of academicians and health care providers who come into a community for their own purposes, fulfill their task, and leave. We have made it clear to community leaders that we will maintain a continuous presence as much as possible. Since we don't have students in the summer months, faculty members have maintained those ties by doing blood pressure clinics at some sites and attending community festivities. Additionally the same group of students will return to the same community both junior and

senior year. This enables community leaders and clients to become familiar with the students and faculty and to build trust. It enables students to
build on previous experiences and their knowledge of community
resources and cultural considerations in care delivery.

Discussions with community leaders also revealed the distrust minority communities have with health care providers who impose their own
health care agenda when they come into a neighborhood. Gaining a better understanding of that distrust and knowing that many programs
offered to minority communities have not been successful led us to our
second philosophical tenet. We feel it is vital to allow neighborhood leaders to determine the needs of the community so that opportunities for students are neighborhood led and are not imposed from the outside by
faculty or students. At the beginning of each clinical rotation the students
plan their agenda based on projects the neighborhood leaders have identified as taking priority. Sometimes it is a new project; often it is the continuation of a project the previous clinical group had initiated.

The third philosophical tenet is that cultural awareness leads to providing culturally competent nursing care and that is it an important part
of the nursing curriculum. Prior to the implementation of our neighborhood based clinical education, a relevant part of the Family Nursing course
had been for students to research different cultures for group presentations. We knew we wanted to continue having the students gain knowledge about different cultures in our neighborhood nursing clinical and to
broaden that knowledge to make it a foundation for their clinical experience. American International College has a strong mission statement on
globalization. In relation to that, the Director of the Division of Nursing as
well as faculty decided that part of the mission of the division is to promote cultural competency as awareness of health care needs of minority
populations living in the various neighborhoods of our city. There are rich
opportunities to interact with persons from other cultures in Springfield
in every health care setting. Our objective is that students will learn about
the prevailing culture in the neighborhood by gathering information from
both community members and academic sources using the Cultural
Functional Health History as a guide. They will then apply that knowledge to begin to ensure culturally appropriate interactions and interventions with clients.

Integration of Neighborhood Clinical Experience

The students are introduced to health promotion and cultural awareness
concepts in nursing foundational courses in the sophomore year. [Refer
to Table 7-1.] Fall semester junior year is devoted to Adult Medical

Surgical Nursing including an acute care clinical experience. In the hospital setting, as students care for patients from many cultural backgrounds, they are sensitized to the need for both cultural competence and health promotion.

The first neighborhood experience is introduced as one of three clinical rotations in spring semester junior year in conjunction with the Family Nursing course and a Family Assessment course. These courses provide students health promotion concepts with childbearing and childrearing families and with formal teaching learning principles. The two major project requirements in the neighborhood clinical are completing the Cultural Functional Health History and a teaching project with clients in the assigned neighborhood.

Both of these projects incorporate concepts from previous nursing courses as well as current nursing courses. The Cultural Functional Health History broadens the scope of the functional health assessment. Students progress from assessing a patient in a rehabilitation facility or nursing home in the sophomore year to adult acute care patients in the junior year, and finally pediatric and maternity patients and families. The functional health patterns now are applied to a specific culture to guide the student's learning and to make cultural knowledge relevant to the nursing process. These cultural concepts, developmental considerations from Developmental Psychology and the Family Nursing course, and teaching learning principles from the Family Assessment course, as well as nursing theory from previous nursing courses, are all applied to the formal teaching projects each clinical group does in the neighborhoods.

The teaching projects are based on community needs identified by neighborhood leaders and are often serendipitously discovered by the students themselves in their interactions with neighborhood residents. The students have taught health, hygiene and basic nutrition to a group of African American children with physical, cognitive, and behavioral disorders. They taught First Aid and safety courses to groups of Hispanic Boy Scouts. Students working with the Vietnamese population were asked to teach about Hepatitis C, dietary considerations associated with high blood pressure, and osteoporosis to the community elders. The juniors also participated in weekly blood pressure screenings within the three neighborhoods, various health fairs throughout the city, and the Ronald McDonald city-wide immunization initiatives. In all of these endeavors students were applying didactic material from their nursing courses.

In the fall of senior year, students return to the same neighborhood for the Community Nursing clinical experience. During this rotation, students make individual home visits in conjunction with a visiting nurse association. They also write a formal community assessment paper applying didactic material from the Community Nursing course. The students

TABLE 7-1 American International College
Division of Nursing—Curriculum Plan

Freshman Year		
Semester 1	Anatomy and Physiology	4
	Intro to General Chemistry	4
	English Composition	3
	Intro to Sociology	3
	Physical Education	1
Semester 2	Anatomy and Physiology	4
	Microbiology	4
	English Composition	3
	Introduction to Psychology	3
	Physical Education	1
Sophomore Year		
Semester 1	Pathophysiology	3
	Introduction to Professional Nursing	2
	Public Speaking	3
	Business Application of Microcomputers	3
	Developmental Psychology	3
	Math for Medication	1
	Physical Education	1

(continued)

continue their previous neighborhood involvement with blood pressure and glucose screening clinics and teaching projects. Instead of one teaching project per clinical rotation, the senior students may do weekly teaching projects.

During spring semester senior year, students have the opportunity to return to their neighborhood as their clinical leadership experience in the Nursing Leadership course. During this experience, students become more closely involved with neighborhood health providers and community leaders. One of the students who is a single dad worked with a group of men in the African American community teaching parenting skills.

Leadership students in the Hispanic neighborhood brought the need for local immunization clinics to city officials. An ongoing leadership project is the development and implementation of an Asthma Environmental Screening Tool that helps families to assess the home environment for asthma triggers. Students integrate didactic material from the Nursing Leadership course as they develop and write formal proposals and a for-

TABLE 7-1 *(continued)*

Semester 2	Literature	3
	Fundamentals of Nursing Practice	6
	Pharmacology and Nutrition	3
	Humanity Elective	3
	Statistics	3
	Physical Education	1
Junior Year		
Semester 1	Adult Medical Surgical Nursing	9
	Nursing Research	3
	Humanity Elective	3
Semester 2	Family Centered Nursing	10
	Family Centered Nursing Process	2
	Social Science Elective	3
Senior Year		
Semester 1	Community Focused Nursing	6
	Psychiatric/Mental Health Nursing	6
	Social Science Elective	3
Semester 2	Complex Medical Surgical Nursing	6
	Nursing Leadership	6
	Trends and Issues in Nursing	3

mal change paper. They also apply leadership principles as they mentor junior students in the neighborhood setting.

ASPECTS OF NEIGHBORHOOD-BASED EDUCATION
SELECTION OF THE NEIGHBORHOODS

The city of Springfield has a population of over 157,000 persons with a wide range of cultural and ethnic backgrounds. The city is divided into nine separate neighborhoods. Groups of people of the same race and ethnicity can be identified on the basis of neighborhood boundaries. As the faculty developed the neighborhood-based clinical program, Springfield's largest minority populations of African American, Hispanic and Vietnamese were identified as our focus groups within the city neighborhoods of Mason Square, Forest Park, and the North End.

Mason Square Neighborhood

The Mason Square neighborhood was readily identified as a focus area because this neighborhood is home to the college. The faculty felt it was very important to make strong outreach efforts in the community closest to home. This neighborhood has approximately 5,000 residents primarily of African American descent. Initial outreach in this neighborhood began with linkages to the Neighborhood Health Center. This center is affiliated with BMC, and the relationship with the BMC Cultural Awareness Committee, as well as one of our faculty members close association with the facility and the director, assisted in the planning stages.

The first group of students spent part of their time assessing needs and providing health education to clients who came to the center for health care. The students focused their attention on those clients in the waiting rooms rather than working with a specific provider. This was at the request of both the medical and nursing directors who earnestly wanted to meet the needs of the clients in providing education and outreach. Clients spent long periods of time waiting to be seen by providers or for tests allowing time for students to meet informally with them.

Students were also assigned to explore the neighborhood and to identify resources that were available and used by neighborhood residents. The students and faculty quickly became aware of more appropriate sites for the application of neighborhood nursing interventions.

Students identified the Martin Luther King Jr. Community Center in the Mason Square neighborhood as a popular resource center for residents of all ages. Programs include comprehensive after-school and weekend youth development activities, athletics, tutoring, college planning, prevention services, and adult education. There is an alternative city high school on the site. Every Friday morning, there is a weekly food distribution program, and emergency food assistance is also provided. The staff at the community center was extremely interested in establishing a link with nurses from the college, particularly since the college is a close neighbor.

The nursing students began to informally visit the recipients during the Friday food program and soon began to provide blood pressure assessments on a weekly basis. This service has now grown to blood pressure screening, glucose monitoring, and medication assessment and teaching, all on an individual basis. Senior nursing students began providing follow-up assessments for those individuals who were identified as high risk for health problems. The goal is to begin outreach to people's homes when hypertension or diabetes is identified as a health problem in order to provide further assessment and education.

Junior students at the Martin Luther King Center were asked to work with children in the after-school program. The ages of these children range from 5 to 16 years. A few of the groups included children with physical, developmental, and/or behavioral disorders. The staff identified many stressors within the children's home environments. The students were asked to provide health teaching to these groups of children on a wide range of topics. The students first spent time with the children to assess their developmental level and learning needs. Initial projects focused on safety issues, but other student groups began to work on more complex areas such as self-esteem and self-awareness. During this process the faculty developed a formalized agreement with the agency to provide health promotion to their clients across the life span.

Forest Park Neighborhood

The second focal neighborhood, Forest Park, has approximately 5,000 to 6,000 Vietnamese American residents. The Vietnamese American Civic Association was identified as a key community agency. Faculty were familiar with the staff through contact with the BMC Cultural Awareness Committee. The association with this organization was immediately formalized through a written contract once it was recognized that the residents valued the services of this agency.

The Vietnamese American Civic Association (VACA) provides services to Vietnamese refugees and other immigrant groups living in the Springfield area. Available services include ESL (English as a second language) classes, interpretation, translation, social services, and U.S. Citizenship classes. There is a very active youth program offering academic tutoring, recreational activities, tobacco control and prevention, and promotion of a positive cultural identity. The agency's Elder Health Program has health education as a primary focus including prevention of diseases such as hypertension, diabetes, osteoporosis, hepatitis, and HIV. Health care providers from the area are invited to provide information on health-related issues and services. There is a monthly Health Resource Day for the elders which has a consistent attendance of 30 men and women.

The students' first contact with residents in this community was during the Tet celebration. Students and faculty helped with the preparations for this event and attended the day-long celebration at a local high school. They assisted the members of the BMC Cultural Awareness Committee in blood pressure screening and disseminating health care materials. They were then invited to provide blood pressure screening and health care education at the monthly Health Resource Day for the community elders. Students also visited with the children in the after-school program. Student clinical activities have slowly grown as acceptance within the community has increased. Senior students, after two years of contact with the community, were requested to provide HIV education to young males. This privilege only occurred once the level of trust had been established gradually between the neighborhood and the AIC faculty and students.

Brightwood Riverview Neighborhood

The final neighborhood selected was in the North End, specifically the Brightwood Riverview section of Springfield. This community is extremely active with many thriving community agencies. The residents are primarily Hispanic Puerto Rican Americans, very proud of their neighborhood and its accomplishments over the years.

Initial contact was made with the Spanish American Union through their involvement with the BMC Cultural Awareness Committee. The Spanish American Union provides Latino health education, training, and advocacy. Efforts were made to formally integrate junior students into GED classes to provide health education. Here again, once the students began to explore the community, we ventured away from our original alliances as we discovered more applicable opportunities.

As the first rotation of students in this neighborhood was gathering its community resource information, they researched the New North Citizenship Council. When the staff at this agency learned of the college's interest in working in the community, they asked to speak to faculty and introduced us to an outreach worker who was interested in providing more health care services in one of the housing complexes she was involved with.

Serendipity again played a part in our very successful alliance with the Edgewater apartment complex in the Brightwood Riverview section of the North End. This apartment complex has a 10-story building along with many townhouses, housing nearly 500 families. Most of the residents of the high-rise are elderly. Families with more than two children live in the townhouses for safety reasons. This neighborhood is isolated from the rest of the North End and the city by a state highway and a land bridge. It is further isolated from the next neighboring community by the Connecticut River. Most community services including grocery stores are located far from this isolated neighborhood.

The faculty established an informal working relationship with the outreach workers in this apartment complex, and students began to focus their clinical practice in this area. Once again, blood pressure screening clinics were initiated and held twice a week. These clinics have evolved to offer glucose screening and medication counseling. Due to the nature of this ethnic group, these clinics have grown into a form of socialization for the residents. Contact has grown into follow-up with residents in their apartments when a problem is identified. Links have also been established with the Boy Scouts in this area, and students have provided numerous teaching projects with these eager participants.

BRIDGES BETWEEN THE NEIGHBORHOODS
AND THE COLLEGE

All of the early links with the neighborhoods were facilitated or begun from the affiliation with the BMC Cultural Awareness Committee. Once student and faculty assessment of the neighborhoods began, other community leaders were identified and linkages with these agencies were established. The students themselves established many of these bridges as they researched their community assessment assignment. The students became aware of ways to provide health care within these agencies as they met with agency staff and were very interested in planning projects. One group of students researched an agency that provided schooling and services to pregnant adolescents and young moms in the Mason Square area. They asked the director if there was a service they could provide and then taught a class on infant development and parenting.

Most of the college's relationships with neighborhood agencies were informal for the first two years, and then finally formalized in contracts. Once the contracts were agreed upon, the relationship was strengthened and further clinical opportunities were opened to the students. It was very important to move slowly into each of the neighborhoods, establishing trust and demonstrating reliability and commitment to the residents.

The neighborhoods and cultural groups were selected on the basis of the percentage of the cultural groups in the city and the location. The groups were also selected based on the probability that the students would have contact with clients of this cultural background both as students and as graduate registered nurses. Initially, faculty considered rotating students throughout all of the neighborhoods in order to increase cultural competence. This was decided to be ineffective in that the level of trust between the individual students and the community would not be developed unless there was a consistent relationship over a long period of time. Currently, students are in the same neighborhoods working with residents for a portion of three consecutive semesters.

Roles of Neighborhood Leaders and Residents

One of our initial fears about sending students into the neighborhoods was that the persons they would be working with to provide services would not necessarily be nurses and that they might not have a formal education pertaining to their role in the community. This is true, but both faculty and students alike are continually impressed by the knowledge, the love for their community, the advocacy for clients, and the enthusiasm of the service providers who graciously share their time to mentor both students and faculty. It is equally impressive to see how many different people and agencies are providing some type of health care education or services in our city from many different perspectives.

Community residents have also served as mentors as well as clients. They have taught students about their neighborhood and about their culture. They have pointed out resources as well as situations to avoid. They have helped students become more aware of government services and local politics as well as state and national issues that affect their quality of life and their neighborhood. Each neighborhood is rich in role models for students.

The service providers at each one of our neighborhood agencies have informal connections with the students, but students and faculty alike rely on the providers to give the student direction in their clinical contacts with agency members or residents as well as direction for the formal teaching project. The director of VACA and the caseworker who plans the elder Health Resource Day have been mentors to the students in the Forest Park neighborhood. They take students to lunch in local Vietnamese restaurants, teach about their history and culture, provide information about frequent health problems, teach them culturally appropriate ways to interact with Vietnamese people, invite them to community programs, and given them resource material.

The director usually has information-gathering tasks for the students to do for the community. She has also taken students into homes to consult about health problems. Staff at the center has also provided translating services for student presentation. The neighborhood residents provide the students with their stories about life in Vietnam, their struggle to survive during and after the war, and their immigration experiences. Finally, they are always appreciative for student nursing interventions and teaching presentations.

The North End outreach workers and residents serve in similar capacities. The outreach workers in the Edgewater apartment complex are the main resources for the students. They suggest clinical activities based on neighborhood needs and help to coordinate those activities with the residents. The outreach worker who has spent the most time with the students does not have a formal human service education. His expertise comes from many years of advocating for his people and personally helping them with health care concerns. His political savvy brings another dimension to the students in understanding barriers to health care in a minority community. He has involved students in the process of addressing those barriers by initiating a neighborhood survey the students developed on health and safety issues. He has invited them to be present at policy meetings with the local neighborhood health center, and, together, they worked on advocating for an immunization clinic in the housing complex. He refers students to individual residents with health care concerns for follow-up and advocacy. He has also provided links to community resources that may not be welcomed without a personal reference. He cajoles students out of their preconceived ideas of this formerly high crime area of Springfield and the Puerto Rican culture and reminds them when they are not being culturally appropriate. The students' clients have taught them about the Puerto Rican culture, customs, diet, and the importance of family and religion. Some of the women in the apartment complex even make lunch for the students.

In the Mason Square neighborhood our formal alliance is with the director of the Martin Luther King Jr. Community Center. She identifies areas for the students' clinical experiences based on the needs of the center. Students and faculty then work under the direction of specific service providers. The social workers in the after-school program identified the groups of children they wanted the students to work with and the ideas for teaching projects based on their assessment of the children and their needs. They were very clear in addressing appropriate behavior of the student nurses and inappropriate teaching content with the various groups of children who have social problems and/or developmental, behavioral, and cognitive disabilities. The principal of the alternative high school also served in a similar capacity, identifying learning needs, helping to incorporate appropriate content and behavior when teaching a group of adolescent males. It reinforced pediatric nursing content as well as formal teaching learning principles. It also provided the nursing students with positive outcomes from their interventions with the school children and adolescents.

Residents of the Mason Square area have also been invaluable resources for the students. The first group of students in the Mason Square area was fortunate to have an elderly African American gentleman conduct a tour of the neighborhood for the students. This man has an avid interest in the history of Springfield, especially the area around the college. He brought his collection of old postcards of the area and artifacts from the time of slavery to illustrate his talks. He purposely dressed in old clothes to teach students about making instant judgments about people. After hearing about the history of the area, the students and a faculty member would take an automobile tour with this gentleman pointing out the local historical landmarks, the neighborhood changes, and resource facilities the students should be aware of. The tour would end with lunch in a local family restaurant with a typical Southern meal. Everyone in the restaurant knew our tour host and welcomed the students because of this association. This introduction to the neighborhood always gave the students a new appreciation of an area of the city many have previously been fearful of entering. They had a new understanding of the history,

the people, and the vast amount of resources available to the neighborhood residents.

Role of the College Faculty

Three full-time faculty members volunteered to initiate the neighborhood
clinical experience. These faculty members had been strong advocates for
a broader community clinical experience and were aware of the opportunities available in Springfield. The two junior faculty members taught the
15-week Family Nursing course in the spring. The course coordinator's
background is in maternal/newborn nursing in an acute care setting. She
taught that content and had also rotated the junior students through a
community clinical experience at Head Start. Her background in nursing
administration made her keenly aware of the changes in health care
delivery and the need to give our students clinical experiences outside
the hospital setting.

The other junior faculty member's practice area is acute care pediatrics.
She came with knowledge of Springfield through prior volunteer civic and
church involvement with various city-wide agencies and had also worked
with resettling a Vietnamese refugee family. The third faculty member has
a background in gerontology. Her practice area is community and public
health nursing. She brings rich and varied experiences in that practice area,
strong ties to the African American community, and the perspective of a
woman of color. She teaches Family Assessment to the juniors in the spring
semester and Community Nursing to the seniors in the fall semester.
Adjunct clinical faculty have been persons with both a community nursing background as well as maternal/child.

Faculty members have established strong relationships with the residents and staff at the various community agencies. Faculty has provided
coverage for ongoing health assessment clinics during the semester breaks
and summer months in order to promote trust within the community.
Faculty members have attended various community and cultural functions
bringing family members along to enjoy the festivities. Faculty members
have also established relationships with other city-wide community agencies in an effort to promote AIC as a provider of health education and nursing care. The responsibilities for the involved faculty have increased each
year due to requests from the community for input and assistance.

The faculty has also maintained an alliance with the BMC Cultural
Awareness Committee. This committee meets every other week. The faculty members have taken turns to be present at the meetings and to participate in the tasks of the committee. Part of their role is to be a liaison
between the neighborhoods and the committee. Neighborhood health care
concerns are brought through the committee to the hospital administra-

tion. Faculty members have suggested speakers for cultural inservices at the hospital and have brought students to attend the presentations. Committee members, nursing faculty, and students have exchanged cultural knowledge and community resource information to positively effect health care delivery. Nursing students, faculty and committee members have participated together at community gatherings. A banner was made to signify this relationship between the committee and the college and is displayed at community health fairs.

Faculty responsibility to students follows a typical role of clinical faculty. The faculty member introduces the students to the course objectives and requirements. Then the students are introduced to the neighborhood site and to any service providers who may be present. Faculty will provide the students with background information about the agency and the provided services, some information about the neighborhood and the residents, and some information about the culture. Faculty will guide students in planning their clinical rotation and each day's events and then allow the students to explore the neighborhood on their own while meeting the clinical objectives. The faculty is always available by beeper and by cell phone. Students are expected to inform faculty of their plans for the day and where they will be.

In the junior year, two faculty members rotate between the three sites to be a resource to the students and to link with the service providers the students are working with. The junior faculty also supervises senior leadership students and facilitates their role in the neighborhood. In the senior year, there has been a faculty member available for each site depending on the student enrollment. In senior year faculty needs to be available for supervising home visits. Faculty serves to facilitate the interaction between the students, the service providers, clients, and other healthcare resources. Most importantly, faculty models the nursing role in the neighborhood.

Students submit weekly journals accounting for their clinical time and processing their experiences. Faculty is responsible for reading, grading the journals, and addressing specific issues with students or service providers brought forward in the journals. The faculty also works with the students in the development of their formal teaching project and evaluating them during a rehearsal session as well as during the actual presentation. The teaching projects are also submitted in a written format which faculty reviews and grades. The junior students present their cultural assessment to each other at the end of the semester. The faculty facilitates these presentations and evaluates the students. Senior Leadership course requirements are also evaluated by the junior faculty supervising those students. Clinical faculty in the senior Community Nursing course is responsible for evaluating student written work and presentations as well as supervising home visits. At the end of each clinical rotation the faculty member will meet with individual students for their course evaluation.

Role of Students

Students are assigned to a neighborhood in the spring semester of the junior year and then return to this community for the fall of senior year. A number of students also choose the neighborhood for a voluntary leadership experience in the spring of senior year. Students are placed into clinical groups on the basis of strengths and weaknesses for a balanced group. Some of the attributes we consider are student's ability to relate to clients in a comfortable manner, ability to be self-directed, degree of assertiveness, previous life-experiences in similar situations, and the ability to work cooperatively in groups. Students from the same ethnic or cultural background are usually placed in that neighborhood. This is done for various reasons, the most important one being that community leaders have requested it. These students gain insight into their cultural or ethnic background and a new appreciation of their neighborhood if they are from Springfield and are excellent role models for the children within the neighborhood. We have found that clients have been very excited to see student nurses from their neighborhood or ethnic background trying to learn more about the neighborhood and culture and to deliver health care. In our three neighborhoods elders are revered and are a source of wisdom to the younger generation. This makes for a unique relationship of mutuality and respect between the client and student nurse.

The initial orientation of junior students to the neighborhood is usually by the faculty and is then continued by seniors students, by community leaders, and finally by the students' independent exploration of the neighborhood in small groups. The most successful orientations have been from some of the senior students and from neighborhood leaders. Junior nursing students come to the neighborhood clinical with great discomfort over the limited amount of structure, the required independence, and misconceptions about the neighborhood and culture. Senior students quickly dispel much of that discomfort by talking about their own fears as juniors, and then by describing the personal growth that has taken place as they discovered unknown attributes within themselves and the community. One senior nursing student told the juniors "This is the best clinical experience of all" because of the independence and the creativity. He went on to tell the students that he had found his niche in nursing in the community and public health area and now plans to attend graduate school to continue his knowledge development. That student led an enthusiastic tour of the neighborhood. He continued his work in the community by choosing it as a leadership experience as did some of the juniors he oriented. To facilitate the students' independent community orientation, we adapted "The Environmental Survey" from Teaching Nursing in the Neighborhoods (Matteson, 1995, p. 195). Students walk around the neighborhood as well as drive around the larger community. This assignment is completed the first week of the clinical rotation to increase the students' comfort level in the neighborhood. Students are also required to research a community agency noting the services provided, funding, use by the neighborhood cultural group, and barriers to providing care to that group as well and facilitating forces. Both of these assignments have produced those serendipitous encounters leading to further relationships between the college and the community such as neighborhood medical centers, the WIC program, and the Springfield Department of Health and Human Services. We also ask students to visit the Massachusetts Prevention Center the first week of clinical. This agency provides a multitude of health care teaching resources and pamphlets for client use. The orientation to the community culminates with the Cultural Functional Health History. Students obtain much of this information through their interviews with community leaders and community residents. These junior year experiences prepare students for the community assessment in the senior Community Health Nursing course.

Student neighborhood responsibilities include the periodic health care screening clinics, presentation of a formal teaching project on topics suggested by the service providers in the community agencies, and following through on other projects the providers have requested. They are in the neighborhood for a period of four to seven weeks depending on the semester for two consecutive six-hour days. Students need to be flexible about their clinical time depending on the meeting times of the groups they are involved with. Students often spend extra time researching their cultural group and planning their formal teaching projects. In addition, weekly students must submit a newspaper article about their neighborhood, the ethnic or cultural group or a health care issue that impacts their assigned neighborhood.

To maintain student continuity in a neighborhood, students research health care needs significant to that neighborhood and then plan projects in conjunction with neighborhood leaders. These projects will be acted upon by the incoming clinical groups or by the same group the next semester they return to the neighborhood. Students feel they are making a contribution to neighborhood health in this manner and look forward to the continuation of their project. Student responsibilities to the college include meeting their course objectives in a professional manner while being accountable for their time in the neighborhood clinical and their clinical assignments. At the end of the junior semester, the students present their experiences and their Cultural Functional Health History. This is a festive occasion for students and faculty including cultural dress, foods, and artifacts. Some of the groups are very creative in their presentation including video or slide presentations of their neighborhood. The pride in their neighborhood and clinical accomplishments are evident. The enthusiasm is catching and all the students learn about the different neighborhoods, resources, and culture as well as each other.

Evaluation of the Neighborhood Clinical Experiences

A neighborhood-based clinical education experience has ramifications for student and faculty learning as well as the health and well-being of the people of the neighborhoods. Evaluation must be multifaceted and ongoing with input and analysis from all partners.

Benefits to the neighborhood can be looked at and measured in a variety of ways. Clearly, by the end of the first semester senior year, the students have done a significant amount of teaching. Teaching has occurred with various age groups across the life span. Students have worked with teen moms on topics such as normal growth and development, discipline and toddlers, stress reduction, and exercise. Adolescent males requested information on sexually transmitted diseases and substance abuse. Boy Scouts wanted information on safety and First Aid, and children in an after-school day care program were provided information about various topics including safety issues, hygiene, and nutrition. Clients have received information they have requested and that they will find useful in their daily lives. It is expected that these motivated learners will are now better equipped to be informed decision-makers and consumers related to their own health and health of their loved ones.

All formal teaching projects have an evaluation component that must be developed and utilized. Short-term, client-centered objectives are the bases of some type of evaluation format. In general, short-term outcome evaluations demonstrating knowledge gained at the end of one or several teaching sessions have been successful in that clients have demonstrated learned knowledge. Long-term evaluations, through ultimate behavior changes for example, have been more challenging. Senior students and faculty continue to have ongoing dialogue about how to follow up on long-term evaluations. In the Hispanic community students became extremely concerned about a significant number of clients with high blood glucose readings. These students have incorporated multiple interventions based on the date collected over time. As a result, some clients have become more aware of their average blood glucose numbers. Other clients have received weekly, individualized teaching resulting in increased knowledge about their diabetes. Some clients have received home visits with home assessments related to diabetes concerns and connections have been made to family members and health care providers.

Another outcome of the ongoing diabetes follow-up has been increased social interaction of older adults who had previously described feeling isolated and separate. This data finding has been consistent from three years of student assessment projects. The senior students established a "social hour" at the site and clients were encouraged to come with questions and brown bags with their medications. Several women began to attend on a regular basis along with a few men. These individuals are primarily single and retired. All have gained general and individual health information, but equally important, all have used this time to interact with others. Story telling and sharing of life experiences has occurred. At the end of one clinical rotation, one of the participants made lunch for the students as her way of thanking the students for getting her "out of the house" and helping her with medical concerns.

Another ongoing project which brings benefits to the neighborhood is the student participation in the ESL (English as a second language) program at VACA. The clients are predominately Vietnamese Americans and the ESL program has been in place for several years. Initially, the students simply assisted the instructor with the lessons planned during the clinical days they were on site. Students consistently attended the classes and worked one on one or in groups with ESL clients following the instructor's lead. Eventually the students developed and taught short sessions within the ESL classes that incorporated health-related topics.

The students have just completed the third consecutive semester of involvement in the ESL program. The first semester senior students now teach the second hour of the ESL program on their clinical days. They plan a health curriculum for the length of the community clinical experience. One semester, the topics revolved around nutrition, food groups, and the Food Pyramid. That semester, the students included a field trip to a local supermarket with the ESL clients. Another semester, the students taught about body parts and various health and illness-related problems. This ongoing experience has provided a wonderful opportunity for the students to get to know the ESL clients, build trust, and begin to work on culturally competent skills. At the end of the clinical rotations, students have planned small celebrations with the clients and handed out Certificates of Completion as indications of success. Over the weeks warm relationships have emerged between the students and clients. Students have written in their weekly journals about their growing appreciation of the immigrant experience and the harsh realities from which many of the clients have come. A rewarding consequence has been the strengthened relationship with the site director and staff. This has resulted, in part, from the good work the students are doing in the ESL program, the conscientious intent to follow up on all interactions, and the consistency of our presence at the clinical site. The hallmark of this growth in trust led to an invitation by the administrator to work with a group of adolescent males from the community in an AIDS Awareness program this last fall semester. Our students planned a two-hour session with multiple teaching strategies utilized. The 25 teen males were actively involved in the class; they asked pertinent thoughtful questions and initiated lively discussion throughout the session. The trust that we were able to continue to build on eventually resulted in the invitation to work with a segment of the youth population. Faculty and students have been honored and pleased to gradually become a larger part of the activities of this community.

Maintaining the integrity of the fundamental definition of commitment has been important in this community and the other two communities with which our program is involved. A city-wide activity the students participated in was the Ronald McDonald Immunization Initiatives. The students were aware of the low infant and preschool immunization rate in the city. During the first semester of teaching nursing in the neighborhoods some of the clinical groups took on the dissemination of immunization information a part of their teaching projects. Here again, serendipity had an important role. Students in the Mason Square area researched the statistical rates and the use of the local neighborhood health center by neighborhood families for childhood immunizations. They distributed information in local stores, including McDonalds, beauty parlors, the library, and places young mothers might frequent. They knew of the importance of the church in the African American community. In fact, one of these students even counted the number of churches in the neighborhood and arrived at 40. They visited as many churches as possible with information about the importance of immunizations and the place and times for free immunization clinics. In one of the churches they were introduced to a woman who administers a daycare center in the church for adolescent mothers so they could attend school or work. Part of the mother's contract with the agency in return for childcare is to attend parenting classes held at the center. The administrator was always on the alert for teaching resources and she asked the students if they could provide an educational program for these moms on childhood immunization. Needless to say, the students were overjoyed to be able to provide this service through a chance encounter. The following year the junior faculty met with the director of Partners for a Healthier Community through another chance meeting as we tried to follow-up on the immunization initiative. Partners for a Healthier Community in Springfield is an umbrella organization with funding from United Way, BMC, and some area business organizations. Their role is to facilitate and coordinate health care initiatives that are already in place through the use of experienced persons and monies. They were interested in being involved in the Ronald McDonald Immunization Initiative and needed enough people to coordinate the activities. This was a nice fit between the nursing students and the community agencies. The faculty met frequently with the leaders from the many community agencies who were involved, and they took part in the planning with the students. The McDonalds restaurants were located in two of our three neighborhoods. It was important to have many activities planned that would draw families. The nursing students passed out health care information, did face painting and worked with Safe Kids on bicycle safety. These events drew city and state officials including the city Commissioner of Department of Public Health and Human Services as well as the state Health Commissioner. Actual immunizations were not given at the sites, but screening was done and appointments made with health care providers with prizes awarded for both participating in the screening and then at the actual appointment.

The health of the larger neighborhood benefits as individuals are cared for by nurses who, as students, learned about persons in the context of their neighborhood and their culture, nurses who learned how to gather information about and access neighborhood resources, and nurses who learned that successful interventions need to be client led.

Benefits to Student Learning

Students are clearly able to articulate and demonstrate degrees of cultural competence by the end of the two to three semesters of neighborhood based clinical experiences. During the second semester of junior year, the students gather data in a variety of ways to learn about the cultures of interest. Students gain improved research capabilities through literature searches. They also hone interviewing skills by gathering cultural perspectives from clients within the culture for the project. It is viewed as a culminating activity for the semester, and students demonstrate gained knowledge and great creativity when presenting to class and faculty. Various cultural foods are shared and the general climate is one of celebrating diversity.

Another benefit is that students learn where to find educational resources to enhance their teaching. They gain an appreciation of the scarcity of culturally appropriate resources such as visual teaching aides, including videos and pamphlets in the appropriate language, and that includes cultural considerations. As a result, each class has discovered all the artists and "budding artists" and utilized their skills when teaching various populations.

First semester senior students develop the skill of writing and implementing detailed teaching plans that incorporate proposal writing con-

cepts. Once again, students incorporate cultural considerations throughout their teaching interactions with clients in the community. Budget information (small amounts of money are spend during the course of teaching)
is a new area that seniors are expected to include in their written work.

For the junior students this is the first clinical experience where students are practicing more independently. The faculty travels between sites
and is available by beeper and cell phone, but are not always on site when
problems develop; therefore, students have to implement critical thinking.
One encounter was with a non-English speaking Vietnamese woman who
had a glucose screening done at the food distribution site. Her blood glucose level was 39. The students got her some orange juice and food, had
her sit down, and rechecked her 40 minutes later. Her glucose level had
risen and she was feeling well enough to leave.

The students have also learned the importance of evaluation of their
nursing interventions. They have had to reach deep into their knowledge
of human development, including child development, their creativity, and
their ability to think critically. The students who worked with the after-
school groups in Mason Square developed creative board games to evaluate their health teaching. With each correct answer relating to the health
teaching, the school child was able to move his marker on the game. If the
answer was incorrect the marker was moved back a few spaces. The children enjoyed the game, verified that learning had taken place, and
remarked to the faculty member that they "really had fun with the student
nurses!" The nursing students working with the alternative high school
students asked the students to write their questions about sensitive adolescent health care concerns on index cards at their initial meeting. They
then used those cards to plan their teaching. After the teaching session the
students again distributed index cards with questions for the students to
answer as part of their learning evaluation. These interventions led to
lively discussion and participation from all of the class members including the teacher and principal.

Students have also learned to work together in their individual groups
and to pass along ongoing projects, ideas, and insights to the incoming
clinical group. These are important attributes they will be able to bring to
any clinical setting. The ability to work together in groups has been one of
our biggest challenges as faculty members in guiding the students.

Students have also become aware of social and governmental forces that
shape health care. They became aware of the lack of dental care and a phar-
macy in the North End neighborhood and have explored avenues to sup-
ply dental care and affordable medications for the residents. They have a
better understanding of the types of services that are or are not covered by
insurance companies and Medicare or Medicaid. They want to know why
government agencies such as WIC don't provide more substitute food

products and teaching for minority groups who are lactose intolerant after infancy and would not include milk or milk-based products in their diet. They have been involved with the WIC staff in those discussions.

Students have learned how to access and work with community health resources and the importance of multidisciplinary health care role. They have learned some of the problems and limitations clients encounter as they access health care resources. They are more cognizant of the barriers to health care that a minority and immigrant population encounter and of the cultural values which keeps them from utilizing the health care system.

Weekly journal entries illustrate the increasing understanding of students working with vulnerable populations. Students consistently document in the last few journal entries about their sadness in leaving the rotation, the importance of other students following up on activities and projects that they have started, and concern about the general well-being of the clients. Some concepts that continually appear throughout the last few journal entries are respect of the clients, commitment to their needs, and satisfaction of the work accomplished with the clients. One student expressed it this way:

> *"I am sad to say good-bye to this group. It is difficult to end an experience that is personally gratifying. By presenting information that, to us, seemed so simple we largely impacted people's lives. The teaching-learning experience held meaning for everyone involved. This has been the most meaningful clinical experience for me yet and I hope others are able to have such a positive experience as well."*

Another student wrote in his last journal entry about "the humbling experience" of hearing the stories of how clients came to live in the United States, fleeing from oppressive governments to internment camps, and eventually finding their way to the United States. The last line of this student's journal stated simply that "this rotation has helped me to come back in touch with my ability to empathize." The historical context of the clients' experiences has drawn out the best qualities in these students, moving them closer to cultural competence in their nursing practice. By the end of the senior community rotation, many students are able to articulate and apply a broadened definition of health into their practice.

Benefits to Faculty

The opportunity of meeting and working with community advocates, outreach workers, and individuals who are engaged and have a history with the community and community groups has been inspiring. These individuals are exemplary role models for faculty members; love for their communities is so visibly evident that it helps to sustain all who work with them. Our program's fundamental premise of commitment to the communities is observed in their daily lives.

The faculty members who have been integrally involved in this curriculum shift to neighborhood-based nursing from the beginning have gained a vast amount of knowledge about these cultures. Affiliation with the Cultural Awareness Committee at BMC has led to the co-sponsoring of multiple workshops and inservices about various cultures. Organizations and institutions within the larger community are now contacting AIC faculty when cultural events and health activities are occurring. Program recognition has also increased which has benefited the faculty, the division of nursing, and the college.

The faculty members who came from an acute care background have been amazed by the opportunities to practice health care in the community. We have increased our knowledge about public health issues and related nursing theory that is brought back to our lectures and into our acute care clinical teaching. Our enthusiasm has been infectious. Other nursing faculty members have begun to investigate the possible movement of other areas of our nursing program into the neighborhoods as well as other divisions within the School of Health Sciences at the college.

FUTURE PLANS

We have started the process of moving the neighborhood-based clinical program into other courses. During the Psychiatric Nursing clinical the students stayed in their same neighborhoods to do a teaching project in an outpatient psychiatric facility while devoting most of their clinical time to inpatient psychiatric nursing. For the most part it was successful. One group project, however, veered from the written outline so, in the future, the groups will rehearse their presentations with a faculty member before presenting them.

In the future we will try to find ways to involve students in the neighborhoods during their Fundamentals course and the Adult Medical Surgical Nursing course. Currently we remain concerned about taking away acute care experience from our current nursing students.

Our faculty would also like to have a full-time faculty member to provide consistency in the neighborhoods throughout the academic year and during semester breaks. Our current method is workable only because we keep an ongoing dialogue concerning the neighborhoods and the students. Another positive aspect is that we each bring a different perspective and different talents that strengthen our program. The drawback is that we don't have the consistency which may be more appreciated in the neighborhood sites and the community at large. Also, when enrollments are high, it is important to have a person who can devote more time to pre-planning and coordination

We would also like to expand our outreach. Our asthma program is in its infancy and bringing that into the other neighborhoods is an identified and requested need in the city. We have a large Russian population in the Forest Park neighborhood and we would like to explore ways to work with them. There are many more programs we could be involved with, both at the Martin King Jr. Community Center and at the Edgewater apartment complex. The service providers at more sites keep requesting more students.

Future plans include expanding our outreach to children in the neighborhoods to provide role models and mentoring. That may include collaboration with other departments in the college to meet neighborhood needs.

We continue to refine our assessment and evaluation tools and to explore ways in which to strengthen the student's group work. The process is ongoing and challenging.

LESSONS LEARNED DURING THIS DEVELOPMENTAL EXPERIENCE

Initial Steps to Positively Engage Faculty with the Division of Nursing

There were numerous factors that helped facilitate our movement into the neighborhoods. Overall was the change in health care delivery that was impacting nursing. We were in the process of a curriculum change to help students quickly adapt to the increased acuity levels in the hospital. We were also aware of the decreased number of clinical placements with hospital downsizing and the growing number of nursing opportunities outside of acute care facilities. We wanted our students to have more experience outside of the traditional hospital clinical settings. Our faculty was ready for change.

Our Director of the Division of Nursing is very supportive, continuing our exploration during Curriculum and Evaluation Committee meetings, and hiring adjunct clinical faculty in the acute care area to free those of us most interested in moving into the neighborhoods to proceed.

We were also fortunate that the college is located in the middle of one of our neighborhoods and to be geographically close to other neighborhoods. The college had already established some outreach programs in the immediate neighborhood. One of our faculty members was a board member of the local neighborhood health center and had been invited by the medical director to participate with students in community outreach. We began to meet with him and the director of nursing to explore their needs and possible opportunities for students. Some of us had strong ties to Baystate Medical Center (BMC) that facilitated our alliance with the BMC Cultural Awareness Committee, and they were eager to link with local nursing schools. We had worked with some of the committee members in the past as staff nurses so relationships had already been established and work could begin.

Although the faculty was supportive, we were concerned about decreasing the amount of time spend in acute care. We were also concerned about adding to our workload in the midst of a substantial curriculum change. Our faculty is small with one member who has a strong community health nursing background. The other two faculty members involved have acute care backgrounds, but in spite of that they brought enthusiasm and a little courage to the endeavor.

DEVELOPMENT OF NEIGHBORHOOD PARTNERSHIPS IN CLINICAL EDUCATION

Activities of the Faculty

Most of our partnerships were developed serendipitously through faculty or student interactions. In two of our neighborhoods our initial partnerships were not appropriate for the type of clinical educational opportunities we envisioned. Both faculty and students were uncomfortable for various reasons, and, through students explorations of neighborhood resources, we were led to more appropriate opportunities. It was awkward to leave the initial sites early in the semester, but it was wise to follow our instincts and do so. The junior students in that first rotation felt angry, but they soon realized at the end of the semester from the other students and during their senior year clinical rotation that the change was positive for all concerned.

One of the deterrents at the neighborhood health center was that the majority of providers did not understand the student objectives. When they realized that the nursing students were not there to settle patients into examining rooms following a medical model, they were aloof and, often times, students were asked to leave the exam rooms. The staff had been prepared for the outreach objectives students were asked to do from the center's director, but affiliation with a large teaching hospital brought many other nursing students, medical assistant students, and medical residents who assumed our students would fulfill traditional roles. It was a confusing situation for staff and students alike.

During the first two years, the junior faculty members were in the community. They worked diligently to establish neighborhood partnerships and bridges to other agencies by attending individual meetings with community leaders and health care providers and by being involved on various committees throughout the city. It was really a crash course in learning who the major players are and how to establish relationships outside of an institutional setting. We were actually fortunate in having a large enrollment in those classes because students also did a lot of leg work in groups of two as they learned about the neighborhood resources and brought that information back to faculty. The process was energizing for both students and faculty because so many providers were interested in what we were doing and expressed an interest to have nursing students work with them. The first year, we had enough students to assign a group each week to help out at dinnertime in a soup kitchen for the homeless. We had hoped to work with the nurses who practice in the local Healthcare for the Homeless agency, but their liability issues would only allow them to accept graduate students who are registered nurses. It was a temptation to overextend our neighborhood outreach because so many opportunities were available.

We are now comfortable in the three main sites we serve in our neighborhoods. That process evolved over three years by moving slowly and gaining trust through commitment. We have formal contracts now at each site. The commitment is nurtured by faculty members who continue to provide volunteer services on a limited basis during semester breaks. Unfortunately, we are unable to have the same full-time faculty members in the neighborhood-based clinical during the academic year because of commitment to other courses. One of our visions for the future would be to have a full-time neighborhood clinical coordinator who would also be available during semester breaks.

Each year the neighborhood faculty members need to reestablish themselves in the community by meeting with the director or outreach worker at each site prior to the start of clinical, catch-up on the changes within the agency including new staff and programs, and establish some plans for the coming semester. We also need to reestablish the level of students and their clinical objectives. It can be difficult for staff who have worked with senior students in the fall who are oriented to the agency, staff, the neighborhood, and the culture from their junior year to begin again with brand new junior students. We have to remind the staff that our expectations and objectives for the juniors are not at same level as for the seniors.

We have also discovered that we need to be very flexible in planning projects or meetings. Numerous times the students have planned teaching projects in conjunction with a service provider which have had to be postponed to another day or shortened because something else took precedence or changed, to be presented to another group. This can be very frustrating for the students, but we nurture our relationships with the agencies by remembering we are there to serve their needs, not our own.

The partnership with the BMC Cultural Awareness Committee is also sustained by active involvement of faculty members on the committee and in the work of the committee. This can be difficult because the committee meets at noon every other week at a time faculty members are usually teaching class. We try to take turns attending the meetings while maintaining close communication with the chair of the committee. The students' outreach into the neighborhoods and knowledge about the residents, health care barriers, and resources have been valuable for the Committee members. The minority groups in our neighborhoods have been distrustful of the hospital and other health care facilities for various reasons. Students and faculty have tried to serve in a small capacity as liaisons.

We try to have the students attend the inservices sponsored by the committee on cultural awareness topics the hospital staff has requested. This often means rearranging a clinical day in the neighborhood and pulling students away from the acute-care clinical setting for an hour. These sessions are also videotaped for the staff, and the college is free to use the tapes with students. The nursing students are always appreciative of the speakers and the information provided, and the faculty members have been grateful for dedication of the committee chair and the committee members in bringing cultural awareness to hospital staff.

Students and faculty members have joined with the committee members in various health fairs throughout the city. Faculty members have also collaborated with the committee chair in poster presentations relating to our joint activities at national and local nursing conferences.

Engaging Nursing Students in the Educational Changes

The first group of students to rotate through the neighborhood-based clinical education was in the midst of an overall curriculum change. We started preparing them for the spring semester during the fall semester as we told them about the exciting possibilities in the three neighborhoods that we planned to work in. We explained the philosophy of our neighborhood-based curriculum and told them that the skills they would gain would be beneficial in any setting they would choose to practice in as well as give them some accomplishments on their resume that may make them stand apart from others. These students were already fearful that they would be unable to get hospital positions because of downsizing, so many were open to explore other aspects of nursing. Faculty members kept talking about the new clinical as much as possible during the fall semester and tried to integrate some of the concepts into the Adult Medical Surgical Nursing course. When spring came, the students looked forward to starting clinical. Our plan was to place the strongest groups possible in those first rotations to get off to a good start and to prepare the way for the next groups.

Other than a total immersion into another culture in an unfamiliar neighborhood, the students' biggest concern was the decrease in the amount of structure they were used to along with the amount of supervision. After their orientation, their first question always was and continues to be "But what do we do?" We have learned it is important to give those junior students definite assignments the first week to give them a sense of direction and security. It is even helpful to give them more than they can get done. We have also learned it is important for them to give a log of their daily activities in their weekly journals to make them accountable for their time. They are also asked to establish goals for each clinical day and what they did to accomplish those goals as well as to set goals for the coming week. At first, the goals are very general but, as they progress through the rotation, the goals become more specific.

Another concern was personal safety in some of the neighborhoods. "My boyfriend" or "my father doesn't want me in this neighborhood." The perception of crime in those neighborhoods is much higher than the actuality. Springfield is fortunate to have community policing, and it has been helpful to have the students meet with the community police to dispel their fears and to learn to move about the city in a reasonable manner. The community police officers are proud of their neighborhoods and the changes they have been able to effect, and the students have been able to realize that they are an asset and a resource.

Finally, students are expected to work in groups and for the first time they receive group grades. Clinical at AIC is pass/fail, and, if a student fails clinical, she fails the whole course. The formal teaching project the juniors do in the neighborhood setting, however, receives a group grade from the Family Assessment course, and the cultural presentations at the end of the summer receive a group grade from the Family Nursing course. Students complained in their journals or to faculty that others in their group were not contributing their fair share to the group projects. Often groups within the same neighborhood would refuse to share information with their colleagues or with the incoming groups because they feared the other groups would receive higher grades on their projects. There were also issues of incompatibility in the approach to tasks or setting congenial meeting times. To address the grade issue we decreased the weight of the group projects in students' overall course evaluation. This past year we also split the grade to award a group grade and an individual grade. We noticed an overall increase in the quality of the projects from this group of students with more coorperation. We also quickly follow up on group issues by trying to have the group members work their problems through independently with faculty direction. If that isn't successful, faculty will meet with the entire group to address the issues. It is important to impress upon the students that the ability to work cooperatively in groups is a skill that is essential in practice, and that sharing knowledge about a community or a projects is just as important as sharing information about a patient they are caring for whether it is among an interdisciplinary team or at report to the oncoming nurse. We have also decided to spend more time on the introduction of group dynamics earlier in the curriculum and to bring those concepts back to students as they are working together in the neighborhoods.

SUMMARY

This chapter began by discussing the attributes of courage and serendipity. Our curriculum change to teaching nursing in the neighborhoods began with a vision and a lot of courage to pursue that vision. We are fortunate to have a supportive director, supportive faculty, and a supportive college administration who urged us to follow our instincts as we applied the Northeastern University model in the city. Our early fears about not having enough for the students to do in the neighborhoods and concerns about which agencies we would work with fell away once we were open to serendipity. Isn't that the real challenge in our nursing profession?

We begin each day in our practice not knowing what will confront us or which resources we will draw on, but we know how to make a quick assessment, prioritize our interventions, be flexible and open to the unexpected, and rely on our knowledge and the knowledge and support of our colleagues. We realize that if we make plans for our day they are sure to change. We also know that if we make goals they may have to be adjusted to meet our objectives. Teaching nursing in the neighborhoods brings that same challenge and the same opportunities to practice and grow.

We made some tradeoffs. It is harder to measure many of the intangible skills students gain in the neighborhoods verses the very measurable tangible skills they are asked to perform in the hospital clinical area. Not every student finds the experience beneficial, but those students are in a small minority. We continue to be pleased by the individual student growth displayed in the neighborhood-based clinical. Most of the student's evaluations are positive, and they look forward to continuing the work they started in the junior year to the senior year. Many of the students have gone on to public health or community nursing, bringing the skills they gained with them. As one of our enthusiastic seniors told the juniors before their first neighborhood clinical rotation, "Community is where it is at! It is the place where you can make your own decisions, be independent, and have the most effect."

REFERENCES

Clark, M. J. (1996). *Nursing in the community* (2nd ed.). Stamford Connecticut: Appleton Lange.

Dresser, N. (1996). *Multicultural manners: New roles of etiquette for a changing Society.* New York: John Wiley & Sons.

Friedman, M. M. (1992). *Family nursing: Theory and practice* (3rd ed.). St. Louis: Mosby.

Gordon, M. (1994). *Nursing diagnosis: Process and application* (3rd ed.). St. Louis: Mosby.

Spector, R. E. (1996). *Cultural diversity in health and illness* (4th ed.) Norwalk Connecticut: Appleton Lange.

8

An International Partnership in Jamaica: The Experience of Hartwick College (New York)

Jeanne-Marie E. Havener and Sharon D. Dettenrieder

> *"I learned how nurses in a third world country perform health care without the resources that the United States has. It's been very interesting on the one hand but frustrating and sad on the other because there just aren't enough basic resources. . . . These factors play a big part in health care performance and that's why primary prevention is so important here. They are so far ahead of us in terms of prevention. The people here really taught me a lot about perseverance. I've learned so many things."*
> (excerpt, Student Journal)

Cultural competency in nursing requires that students and clinicians be skilled not only in knowing but also feeling people's experiences and history. With this sensitivity we may begin to understand the logic of their behavior and gain insight into our own behaviors as we provide care providers" (Clinton, 1996). Through a community-based nursing experience in the neighborhoods of Jamaica, West Indies junior nursing students from Hartwick College in Oneonta, New York learn to recognize the myriad of health-related beliefs and practices that exist among and between different members of a culture and how those beliefs and practices impact upon the health of its people.

This four-week experience exposes students to transcultural concepts and theories, encourages application of cultural assessment in diverse urban and rural neighborhood settings, and assists them to understand the meaning of providing culturally competent care to individuals, families, groups, and communities. Students are exposed to different empirical frameworks to assist them in providing holistic, culturally competent care. Clinical care, provided in diverse urban and rural clinic and community settings, emphasizes therapeutic interventions, health promotion, disease prevention, risk reduction, and health teaching within a unique ethno-cultural environment.

PHILOSOPHICAL TENETS OF OUR CLINICAL EDUCATION

The design of our program is based on a desire to assist students to learn the most that they can about the Jamaican culture within a relatively short time while engaging in relationships of mutual exchange. Faculty do not want students to use clinical sites as a laboratory setting or forum for acting upon clients, particularly in light of their "outsider" and developed nation status. Additionally, it was important to faculty that students be able to see the dynamic synthesis of wellness and illness within the context of the lived experience of the client. It was felt that a community-based program was ideally suited for these dual purposes. In the planning phase support for this pedagogical method was found in *Teaching in the Neighborhoods* (Matteson, 1995).

Preparing Students for the Future

In an increasingly complex and intricate world, it stands to reason that the nurse of the future will care for a growing number of persons from diverse populations. According to Leininger (1997) there is a critical need for transcultural knowledge and competency and that requirement will only increase. The necessity of this knowledge is being influenced by: (a) increasing mobility; (b) growing migrant and refugee populations; (c) an increasing recognition of and respect for cultural identity; (d) the evolution of gender roles; (e) the use of technology, electronic communication, and rapid modes of transportation; (f) revealed instances of cultural conflicts and racism in health and human services; and (g) consumer demands to be viewed in a holistic, transcultural manner (p. 341).

As educators we are challenged to prepare the competent nurse of the future. Cultural competence refers to a complex synthesis of "cognitive, affective, and skill dimensions that motivate nurses to care for diverse individuals, families, and communities" (Degazon & Fielo, 1997; Frei,

Hugentobler, Schurman, Duell & Alioth, 1994; Orlandi, 1992). "Cultural competence is characterized by behaviors, attitudes, and policies that enable effective transcultural interactions. A culturally competent individual or agency honors and respects cultural differences. To be culturally competent requires one to be culturally sensitive and aware" (Fletcher, 1997, p. 13; Clinton, 1996, p. 5). Nursing in the neighborhoods, whether it is in Boston, Massachusetts or Jamaica, West Indies, assists students in the process of becoming competent practitioners.

Determining Components of Educational Process

According to the American Association of Colleges of Nursing (AACN) (1998), components of a liberal nursing education include "professional values, core competencies, core knowledge, and role development" (p. 6). Core competencies include critical thinking, communication, assessment, and technical skills. One of the arguments used against establishing a community-based program is concern that such a program will not allow the student to develop technical skills. While it is recognized that "technical skills are required for the delivery of nursing care" and that the "baccalaureate graduate must be adept at performing skills, . . . that include teaching, delegating, and supervising the performance of skilled tasks by others," it is also recognized that nursing students be able to "apply skills in the diverse contexts of health care delivery" (AACN, 1998, p. 11).

Cultural Competency

Campinha-Bacote (1998) proposed the cultural competence model as a framework for teaching cultural diversity that is particularly useful in a community setting. This model views cultural competence as an evolutionary process comprised of four components: cultural awareness, cultural knowledge, cultural skills, and cultural exposure. Cultural awareness is seen as a deliberate and cognitive process whereby the student becomes aware of his or her biases as well as his or her values, beliefs, life ways, practices, and problem-solving strategies (Campinha-Bacote, Yahle & Langenkamp, 1998; Clinton, 1996). Cultural knowledge is sought as a means for understanding variant cultures including their world views, their responses to medications, and/or treatments and assessment findings. Cultural skill, the third component of this process, includes the ability to perform a cultural assessment. Finally, during the cultural encounter, the student directly engages in cross-cultural interactions with individuals from culturally diverse backgrounds. This experiential knowledge is felt to be foundational to developing culturally relevant nursing interventions (Campinha-Bacote et al, 1998, p. 122–24).

The essence of any professional education lies in the way the students are integrated and taught to practice the discipline. C.A. Shea suggests, that because persons' lives are spent in their community, meaningful nursing education should likewise incorporate experiences in this setting (Shea, 1995). These clinical experiences are said to encourage students to see the "big picture," encounter diversity, and participate in the dynamic synthesis of health care and health care decision-making within the context of the peoples' lives. Experiential encounters in the neighborhoods of rural Jamaica prove worthwhile in terms of meeting these learning objectives.

> *"Every situation has been a learning experience. I learned so much... working in the community and going inside the homes of the people who lived there, made it all real. Just to meet the people, see the types of homes they live in, learn about what they do with their time and money, how they earn their money, the way they live, dress and eat. At times in the clinic, I would get bored, thinking I wasn't "doing" enough . . . now I realize that what I learned was different . . . it was more than I imagined."*
> (excerpt, Student Journal)

In 1991, the American Nurses Association (ANA) published *Standards of Clinical Nursing Practice* which called for nursing to take responsibility for providing culturally and ethnically relevant care. The American Academy of Nursing's publication, *Promoting Cultural Competence in and Through Nursing Education* (1995) pointed out that professional competence must encompass cultural competence and is an integral part of ". . . preparing a competent, humanistic, practitioner" (p. 16). The National League for Nursing (1993) and more recently the AACN (1998) have emphasized the need for schools of nursing to adopt multiculturalism and a commitment to diversity within their curricula:

> *"Human diversity includes understanding the ways cultural, racial socioeconomic, religious, and lifestyle variations are expressed. Baccalaureate graduates must be able to apply knowledge of the effects of these variations on health status and response to health care"* (AACN, 1998, p. 15).

The AACN (1998) calls for clinical experiences that provide the graduate with the knowledge and skills to: "understand how human behavior is affected by culture, race, religion, gender, lifestyle and age; provide holistic care that addresses the needs of diverse populations across the life span; work collaboratively with health care providers from diverse backgrounds; understand the effects of health and social policies on persons from diverse backgrounds; and advocate for health care that is sensitive to the needs of patients, with particular emphasis on the needs of vulnerable populations" (AACN, 1998, p. 15).

Further, the National League for Nursing (1993) advocated that nursing education shift to a focus on community-based programs with an emphasis on health promotion, disease prevention, and risk reduction.

Despite this emphasis on transcultural and community-based nursing, educational preparation continues to emphasize mastery of psychomotor skills, an illness model, Western traditions of care and treatment, and hospital-based nursing care (Kulwicki & Boloink, 1996, p. 41; Shea, 1995, p. 36; Wuest, 1992, p. 90). While educators might agree that critical thinking, communication, assessment, and technical skills are core competencies, it is equally important that nurses develop an understanding of the "bigger picture" or "patterned whole," in order to provide compassionate, meaningful care to others. To achieve this vision of a "patterned whole" nursing students are challenged to understand health as a dynamic synthesis of wellness and illness, plus more (Newman, 1986, p. 12). It is imperative, therefore, for nurses to be equally prepared with the knowledge, skills, and experiences for providing culturally as well as clinically competent care.

INTEGRATION OF COMMUNITY-BASED CLINICAL EXPERIENCES

Antecedents to cultural competency in health care are not known, but it is generally agreed upon that cultural sensitivity and awareness are requisite knowledge (Clinton, 1996, p. 5). To begin the process of becoming culturally aware, first year nursing students at Hartwick College focus on understanding their own cultural heritage and health care practices. Similarities and differences among members of the class are discussed as a beginning framework for understanding other cultures. After being introduced to transcultural nursing theories and concepts, sophomore nursing students are given the opportunity to apply this knowledge through interactive teaching strategies in the classroom and surrounding community. Students are invited to examine their own biases as well as how persons of different cultures socially construct their definitions of health, illness, and health care. Through two activities with people of other cultures, interviews and a group project that centers on health practices and beliefs, students gain insight into how indigenous beliefs and practices might impact upon the nursing care they provide and how the phenomenon of health is socially constructed. These experiences heighten their awareness of the importance of providing care that is culturally appropriate (see Table 8-1).

In essence, the existing curriculum assists students to become culturally sensitive and aware, but it has not allowed them to develop *fully* as culturally competent practitioners. In response to this awareness, a January term was developed to give junior nursing students the opportunity to go off-campus for transcultural learning experiences.

Having achieved some measure of stability in the faculty, endeavors were undertaken to revise the curriculum. Reviewing our curriculum and operating assumptions, we realized that "clinical" was a term reserved for hospital-based experiences while other practicum experiences were referred to as "community experience," "ambulatory care experience," and so forth. These differential definitions created dichotomies that connoted the values of the faculty, i.e., nursing care experiences that occur in settings other than the hospital are of lesser value. It had become clear that we needed to move to a new, broader paradigm of "clinical" that recognized the value and worth of nursing care delivered in diverse settings.

Simultaneous to this beginning paradigm shift came an opportunity to create a transcultural experience for students in Jamaica, West Indies. One of the nursing faculty had traveled to Jamaica on college business and had the chance, while at the University of West Indies campus, to meet with faculty at the Department of Advanced Nursing Education (DANE). In cooperation with the Honorable Syringa Marshall-Burnett, R.N., the current President of the Jamaican Senate and Chair of the DANE, plans were made to develop a transcultural nursing program for Hartwick nursing students.

Another factor that encouraged faculty to embrace this educational initiative included ongoing difficulty in recruiting a faculty member with transcultural expertise, thus necessitating the need for development of this expertise within the existing faculty. Further support for this program initiative was found in the Mission of the college to ". . . educate people who will thrive in and contribute to the world of the future people who are prepared to meet the personal, intellectual, and social challenges of a rapidly changing and increasingly interdependent world" (Hartwick College,1998, p. 5). It is considered an important outcome of the liberal arts experience at Hartwick College that the student develop . . ."a sense of community in a pluralistic context and see one's self as a contributing member of larger communities, with openness and appreciation of differences" (Hartwick college, 1998, p. 14).

Other curricular expectations include "an emphasis on the development of a sense of personal responsibility and focus on service to the community" and "an emphasis on linking theory and practice through use of multiple methods of instruction"(Hartwick College, 1998, p. 30). Additionally, nursing students repeatedly requested opportunities for off-campus programs in the nursing major.

TABLE 8-1 Hartwick College Department of Nursing Curriculum Plan

Yaer	Fall Semester	# Course Units	January	# Course Units	Spring Semester	# Course Units
Freshman	*Biology 110* Human Anatomy & Physiology	1	Elective	1	*Biology 111* Human Anatomy & Physiology	1
	Sociology 105 Intro. to Sociology	1			*Psychology 110* General Psychology	1
	First Year Seminar (CXXI)	1			*Nursing 110* Nursing in Wellness	1
	Elective	1		1	Elective	1
		4				4
Sophomore	*Nursing 231* Nursing in Wellness II	1	Elective	1	*Nursing 233* Nursing in Wellness III	1
	Biology 210 Microbiology	1			*Chemistry 105* Gen'l/Organic/Biochem.	1
	Psychology 201 Life Span Devel. Psych.	1		1	Elective	1
	Elective	1		1	Elective	1
		4				4

TABLE 8-1 *(continued)*

Yaer	Fall Semester	# Course Units	January	# Course Units	Spring Semester	# Course Units
Junior	*Nursing 341* Nuesing in Illness I Sci. 344	1.5	*Nursing 342* Junior Practicum	1	*Nursing 343* Nuesing in Illness II	1.
	Pathophysiology	1	or		Math 108 Statistics	1
	Nursing 345 Pharmacology	1	Nursing 346 Transcultural Nusing	1	Contemporary Issues Seminar (CXXI)	1
	Elective	1		–	Nursing 448	1
		4.5		1	Intro. to Research	–
						4.5
Senior	Nursing 441 Psychosocial Nursing	1	Nursing 495 Senior	1	Nursing 445 Trends & Issues in Prof. Nsg	1
	Nursing 443 Community Health Nursing	1	Independent Practicum	1	Nursing 446 Nursing in Illness III	1
	Nursing 490 Senior Thesis	1		–	Nursing 447 Nursing Management	1
	Elective	1		1	Elective	1
		4				4

Physical Education: 4 Courses (.5 C.U. each)

Nursing	16 C.U.
Pre-requisites	9 C.U.
CXXI Electives	7 C.U.
Free Electives	4 C.U.
Total	36 C.U. + P.E.

Deterrents to program change included difficulty with adapting the transcultural objectives to the existing junior January term syllabus with its acute tertiary care focus. Faculty recognized that the syllabus, as it was constructed, was difficult for faculty and students alike. This awareness allowed faculty to create an alternative, community-based, transcultural nursing course currently offered in Jamaica, West Indies. By creating a separate course, students are now allowed to exercise choice in terms of their learning experience, something that has never previously existed in this major.

Because of the perceived need to give students similar educational experiences, planning for spring semester of the junior year has been altered. Those students choosing the J-term abroad now have more hospital-based experiences in the spring, while those choosing the acute tertiary care focus are given more community-based experiences. This dichotomy speaks to the need for the program to continue to prove itself.

As the program moves forward and students grapple with justifying their choices, faculty find that meeting with all interested parties is important in terms of addressing concerns that, by participating in a non-traditional clinical course, students will be less prepared for subsequent nursing courses.

ASPECTS OF COMMUNITY-BASED EDUCATION

Understanding the Community

Faculty concurred that Jamaica would be an ideal setting for a transcultural experience because of our contacts there and because it is an English-speaking country. Jamaica is a Caribbean nation steeped in the vestiges of European colonization. During colonization, the indigenous AmerIndian populations were virtually exterminated and replaced by a European plantocracy created through the efforts of African slave labor and indentured workers from India, Indonesia, and elsewhere (Momsen, 1993, p. 1). The area has been identified as the "site of a precocious experiment in social engineering and a major crucible from which modern social organizations have evolved" (Hart, 1989).

"Within the Caribbean regional diversity of ethnicity, class, language, and religion there is an ideological unity of patriarchy, of female subordination and dependence. Yet there is also a vibrant living tradition of female economic autonomy, of female-headed households and of family structure in which men are often marginal. . . . The roots of this contemporary paradoxical situation lie in colonialism" (Momsen, 1993, p.1). Given the rich history, culture, and diversity of Jamaica and its well-developed health care infrastructure, it is an ideal location for learning transcultural concepts.

The Jamaican health care system places emphasis on primary health care through the availability of services at the local level through a five-tiered clinic system. Clinics, administered through the Ministry of Health (MoH), provide a variety of health care services to communities where the Nurse Practitioner, Nurse Midwife, and Community Health Aide (CHA) are the major providers of care.

The health problems identified as most significant include: malnutrition; communicable diseases; sexually transmitted diseases; tuberculosis; dental and periodontal illness; hypertension; mental illness; leprosy; cancer of the breast and female organs; and occupational diseases (Leavitt, 1992, p.73).

Facilitating Factors

The Hartwick College program coordinator selected faculty for participation in the program. Selection was based on a shared philosophical understanding about what was to be accomplished, how that could best be accomplished, a willingness to work together, flexibility in meeting goals, and a balance of personal and professional strengths and weaknesses. Because of the particular issues related to taking students abroad and the need to keep student to faculty ratios low, two faculty were sent with 12 students. It was vitally important to the success of the program that the strongest alliance within the group existed between the two faculty. This highlights the need for philosophically aligned world views and a shared understanding of the value of diversity within teaching approaches.

Faculty at DANE, with their inside knowledge of the country, the needs of the population, and available health care resources were invaluable in the planning process. This insider knowledge allowed faculty to explore and plan for the shared exigencies of these two nursing programs. Faculty at Hartwick and DANE were most interested in exploring opportunities for clinical learning that allowed for a meeting of mutual service and academic needs. Additional criteria for site selection included the accessibility of sites as well as use of sites where students would not be competing with others for access to learning opportunities.

PARTNERSHIP BETWEEN THE SCHOOLS

In order to make this program possible, bridges needed to be created and maintained from the neighborhood to academia. The first step in this process was securing a gentlewomen's letter of agreement between DANE and the Hartwick College Department of Nursing. A Jamaican colleague at Hartwick served as a consultant on protocol issues and made possible the first introductions between nursing colleagues at the two schools. Early on in the process it was decided that a contact person was needed from each school in order for program negotiations to solidify.

Faculty are responsible to the college to uphold the spirit and letter of agreement between the two programs and between the UWI and the community centers. Faculty from Hartwick negotiated with faculty at DANE for teaching-learning experiences, clinical affiliations, and opportunities that would support meeting learning objectives and liaisons with whom Hartwick could engage in future program planning. Through a series of phone calls, faxes back and forth, and face-to-face meetings, preliminary plans were accomplished.

Program planning included all of the things that normally go into course preparation including developing course objectives and outcome criteria as well as making food, lodging and ground and air transportation arrangements. Contracts and letters of agreement with the faculty at DANE were used as a means of spelling out needs and responsibilities. Final arrangements for clinical placements were negotiated in face-to-face encounters between Hartwick and DANE faculty after our arrival in the country. As part of the agreement faculty at DANE assisted in making food, lodging, and in-country transportation arrangements as well as gaining our entry into the health care system and neighborhoods. Throughout the process faculty at DANE looked out for our welfare and, at the end of the program, faculty from both schools met to evaluate the program in light of outcomes.

VALUE OF INTRODUCTIONS

In planning such a program it is important to recognize that introductions are a vitally important part of protocol and necessary to establishing positive working relationships. In order for the students to meet objectives, it was important to have acknowledgment of their skills and the trust of the staff at the clinical sites. The DANE faculty went out of their way to bridge this gap. The need for a "bridging person" such as this has also been found to be beneficial by others in setting up transcultural programs (Spitzer, Kesselring, Ravid, Tamir, Granot & Noam, p.324).

Challenges to Program Development

Constraints to program planning include working around issues of time, budgets, politics of the organizations involved, and protocol. Working with an international partner has been both a challenging and rewarding experience. The faculty at DANE were helpful with respect to all aspects of initial planning. Some of our concerns on the planning end have been challenges related to working within a stated budget despite fluctuating exchange rates and unexpected expenses.

Certainly, in planning an international program, one needs to be attentive to regional politics and its influence on the well-being of the group, thus further highlighting the need for cooperative programming with internal contacts. It is important that faculty know the laws of the country related to drug/alcohol use, entry and departure protocols, and cultural norms and values governing conduct. Faculty should bring this awareness into preparation of the students so that any unfortunate incidents might be avoided.

Further considerations in planning an international program include the cultural relativity of time and the differences in academic calendars between international partners. "Soon Come" became a phrase that we learned to live with in the planning and implementation of the program. Putting together a course for the first time in a developing nation with little information regarding costs required a great deal of faith on the part of all participants.

Because of differences in the efficiency and availability of technology between countries, communication can prove challenging. E-mail exists for very few and snail mail is just that. Telephone lines double as fax lines in Jamaica, so faxing is best accomplished during the evening hours. All of this points to the need to plan way ahead of time and be patient, particularly where licensure requirements are a consideration.

Faculty must be shrewd negotiators in terms of finding the best possible prices for travel and lodging. Traveling abroad can be costly. To offset these costs students may have to engage in fundraising efforts, and faculty may seek outside funding opportunities. At the outset, only a preliminary budget may be made. It is, therefore, best to speak to the students in terms of a price range until negotiations are finalized.

Faculty also need to keep students and parents apprised of plans as they evolve. Wherever possible students should be fully engaged in the planning as this provides insights into the people and their country. It can become an integral part of their learning experience.

Additionally, faculty must be cognizant of the fears and misconceptions that students and their family members may have, so, once again, communication is key. Former students may be invited to engage in the process of sharing with prospective students as a means of recruitment and retention in the project. In particular, it is important for students to hear from their peers about the tangible and intangible benefits of such a program. In our case, students have been able to share that they were able to get jobs because their perspective employers were impressed with their experience abroad. In particular, employers have expressed that the students transcultural experience revealed something about them in terms of their flexibility and understanding of diversity.

Throughout the trip, plans are adjusted as deemed necessary. Through contacts that are developed and nurtured, other cultural immersion and clinical opportunities became available. Faculty are charged with responsibility for determining the appropriateness of these opportunities in terms of the student's learning objectives, interests, and budgetary constraints. Accounting was done on a daily basis to maintain an up-to-date sense of our options. Flexibility is a virtue for faculty and student alike.

Negotiations for appropriate clinical experiences are the most challenging part of program planning. Having a baccalaureate nursing program, Hartwick is interested in having students work with similarly prepared nurses. Given the level of practice required in community-based settings, nurses in Jamaica with baccalaureate education or advanced preparation in nursing are more likely to practice in community-based settings. Nurses and the community health care clinics are recognized as pivotal to the health care of the Jamaican people (Catlin, 1996).

Further, it is a concern of Hartwick and DANE faculty that students have an opportunity to see the progressive side of health care in Jamaica as provided by nurses through primary health care initiatives. These initiatives emphasize health promotion, disease prevention, and risk reduction in the setting of limited resources.

Likewise, it is important that students grasp emic and etic perspectives by bearing witness to the "lived experience" of the Jamaican people. The level of care provided in the community and the autonomy of nursing practice evident in the community-based health centers make the community setting ideal for our mutual purposes. The process of choosing sites is based on their established affiliations with the UWI and their needs for assistance.

Urban community sites provide students with an initial exposure to the health practices and issues within the Jamaican culture. Students are engaged in level 4 and 5 (comprehensive) urban community-based centers at the same time that they are participating in health care and cultural immersion activities. These activities include guest lectures from persons living and working within the Jamaican culture and health care system. Lecture topics included health care and political issues in Jamaica, nursing education, the health care system, traditional healing practices, and sickle cell anemia (migration of an illness).

While the students spend only two days at these urban sites, the plan is to continue the affiliation between these two sites and the college. It is hoped that a relationship of mutual exchange will evolve through this continued affiliation.

As with any new endeavor, the presence of the students was initially a case of "more anchor and less steam." The students, however, quickly caught on to the routine and assisted with "hands on" care and teaching. Students participating in the program this year, informed by former participants and faculty, are bringing requested teaching materials that can be used in these settings as a form of continued exchange.

Preparing the Students

Leininger expresses concern about nursing educational experiences that occur within foreign countries or differing cultures with limited health care and transcultural knowledge. Without preparation this has been shown to be "nonconstructive, meaningless and even destructive with pain and shock to students" (1997, p. 342). Leininger (1997) likens this to sending students to care for a person with particular pathology with no prior knowledge of normal physiologic function. Leininger (1995, 1997) further proposes that, to teach transcultural nursing, one must build on a foundation of research-based knowledge, theory, and practice.

Though faculty had engaged students in preparation for the culture that they would be entering, there was recognition among the faculty that these experiences needed to be authenticated and made real in order to be more fully understood. Starting with the urban experiences, assisted students then more easily adapt to their rural clinic experience and, thus, move with less fear of threat out into the neighborhoods. While the students were nervous about stepping out of their initial "zone of comfort," they viewed the urban setting as more threatening than the rural areas. Being from a rural school setting, these fears may have to do with anti-urban bias and idealization of rural lifestyles.

Logan (1995) speaks of our fear of the city as arising out of cultural notions, equating the city danger, anonymity, and lack of social control that is often related to fears and prejudice. Once the students were able to move beyond these fears, however, they exhibited greater confidence and a willingness and openness to seeing and learning more.

> *"In the clinics I did as much as I could-at first I was sort of hesitant about working with the people for fear of not being accepted. However, as time went on and I received more experience, I discovered that the people here are a pleasure to work with. . . . That first day in the clinic in Kingston, I didn't want to give that first immunization because I didn't think the mothers would want a 'white girl' caring for their babies. But through observation, questioning and 'hands on', I now have a totally different outlook"* (excerpt from Student Journal).

The urban experiences stood in sharp contrast to the rural experience, allowing students to compare and contrast differences in health care practices and issues between and among the cultural subgroups. Students were able to readily recognize differences in terms of access to services and risks related to urban versus rural and agrarian lifestyles.

The heart and soul of the nursing education program lay in the rural setting where students spent several weeks in the neighborhoods. The rural setting of Golden Grove in St. Thomas' Parish was specifically selected to provide an opportunity for students to be immersed in an agrarian community. This experience stands in stark contrast to what is experienced in the tourist and urban centers which outsiders most readily identify with Jamaican life.

A Special Neighborhood

The parish of St. Thomas lies in the shadow of the Blue Mountains. Very limited if any tourist infrastructure exists. Towns are few and far between, and life revolves mostly around the plantations and small fishing villages where the work is still performed by canoe and net. The area is one of Jamaica's poorest, as reflected in the living conditions of many of the plantation workers. Conditions have always been harsh here, and the area figured prominently in slave rebellions during the colonial era (Baker, 1996, p. 226).

"Golden Grove is a desperately poor hamlet. Many of the locals are descended from Africans from Sierra Leone who settled on the sugar estates in the decades following emancipation. Corrugated tin and wood huts on stilts are dominated by the landscape of the Tropicana Sugar Estates to the east and the banana plantations to the west. Few dwellings have running water, as the number of people carrying buckets attests. There is a gas station, corner store, school, and numerous churches (Baker, 1996, p. 234).

With the Isaac Barrant Comprehensive Clinic in Golden Grove as a main base, students work with clinic staff providing care in the surrounding agrarian communities. The rural setting allows students to gain a sense of neighborhood community by bearing witness to the norms of reciprocity shared by kinship networks and members of an agrarian community in meeting the daily tasks of living that are at hand. Through nursing in the neighborhoods, students are better able to understand the relationship between the health care beliefs and practices of the Jamaican people, the health care problems and issues of the nation, and the need to provide culturally congruent, meaningful care. Additionally, students are given an opportunity to share something about themselves with others and learn about similarities and differences in values, beliefs, and practices that exist between and among cultures. Finally, through development of a long-term relationship between the neighborhood clinic and faculty of the nursing department, it is hoped that the program will be able to assist local efforts in providing care to this very rural, economically challenged community .

This program allows students the opportunity to provide "hands-on care" in the home and community health clinics. Clinical experiences include well-child, prenatal, postpartal, dental, acute and chronic medical care, family planning, immunization, nutrition, and wound care. Additional clinical experiences include participation in the care of children in an on-site day care center, community health home nursing visits, and working with the Public Health Inspectors as they make on-site visits to assess sanitary conditions in a variety of home and business settings. Students are also able to visit and do formal and informal teaching at local schools and an orphanage.

Within each setting, the senior Public Health Nurses are instrumental in working with faculty to provide students with preceptors. Students work alongside public health nurses, nurse-midwives, community health aides (CHAs), day care staff, and public health inspectors (PHIs) in providing care. Selection of health care providers in the neighborhood is based upon a willingness of providers to work with students and their ability to provide access to neighborhoods. In essence, all of the agency staff at the Isaac Barrant Clinic are open to having students with them. The time spent together is one of great human and professional sharing whereby students and agency staff become genuinely interested in the process of sharing.

In terms of accessing the neighborhoods safely, this linkage is vital. Public health nurses, nurse-midwives, and CHAs are members of the community that they serve.

> *"The students were amazed that the CHA could even find the houses as they may have to go up long winding dirt roads and through wooded areas. CHAs used their connections to find a specific person or where "so and so" was with her new baby"* (excerpt, Faculty Journal).

This insider status allows them access to information that outsiders might not be privy to, not unlike what nurses in community health settings in the U.S. experience. The agency staff give the students access to this insiders' world of privileged information.

By treating nursing students as colleagues, the agency staff assist students in gaining a better understanding of the non-medical determinants and realities of health care in this developing nation. They see the incongruities that exist between the folk and professional health care system and how the health of an individual, group, community, or nation has much to do with their social standing in the larger society.

Agency staff fully participate in the learning experiences of the students. They demonstrate a willingness to assist in finding alternative experiences when planned ones fail; for example, when it rains, home visits aren't made because the dirt roads turn to mud. On one rainy day, the students learned about making supplies out of raw materials and autoclaving supplies and instruments that are routinely purchased or obtained in a pre-packaged form in the United States.

In another instance, there had been an outbreak of violence in the surrounding neighborhood, making it potentially unsafe to do home visits. A gentleman had been killed in the process of burglarizing a home. Because the neighborhoods are composed of strong kinship networks, violence broke out among opposing factions. On this particular day, the neighborhood was cordoned off by police and road blocks had been created by felling trees across the road. This situation negated going out in the neighborhood that day, but created a learning situation whereby staff were able to answer the questions of the students about the meaning of what had occurred. Through this encounter students came to understand the web of complex, affect-laden inter-relationships of mutuality present in this community, community norms and sanctions meted out to those who violate norms.

The use of local drivers assists negotiations on a day-to-day basis as the group interacts with the locals. Throughout the trips drivers function as ambassadors and escorts by making our presence known in the neighborhoods, asking community leaders to watch out for our welfare, negotiating and bartering for services, and further educating us about local protocol and history. As a respected member of the local community, our driver in Golden Grove provided us with invitations to a local church service, a plantation tour, and a tour of a local nursing home—all valuable learning experiences.

Addressing Concerns About Safety

Faculty in the program are responsible for ensuring a safe environment for students. Much time is spent in the pre-planning phase assuaging the fears of students and parents alike. It became clear to faculty, through this process, that, while technically the students were adults, parents were entrusting the faculty to act "in loco parentis." Safety was dependent on the actions of each individual to not invite trouble to the group through naiveté or carelessness. This unique situation created the need for mutually agreed upon rules for the group which were established by the group on the first night of arrival. Infraction of the rules required a group discussion and decision about the repercussions. Safety is a serious consideration to all.

Dealing With Culture Shock

Unlike nursing in the neighborhoods in a community adjacent to one's school, nursing in the neighborhoods abroad has the inescapable challenge of culture shock, 24 hours-a-day, seven days-a-week. Not unlike what Furnham & Bocher (1986) describe, students express, in varying degrees, signs and symptoms of culture shock. The circumstances provoking the culture shock and the individual reactions vary depending on the degree of preparation the student has done, previous experiences with other cultures and travel, the contrasts between home and host environments, and the personality characteristics of the student.

During the first week of the trip some of the common concerns expressed by students at post-conference included: "I am sick of being stared at as if I'm some kind of freak."; "I want to see my boyfriend and my family."; "I wish I could have some macaroni and cheese"; "I'm scared, I don't know what to expect . . . I don't think they (the Jamaicans) like me"; ". . . there are bugs in the shower"; "What do they call this . . . ? . . . food?" (excerpts from post-conference, Faculty Journal)

Culture shock is said to occur in phases: the honeymoon phase; the crisis phase; adjustment, reorientation and gradual recovery phase; and adaptation, resolution and acculturation (Adler, 1975; Rhinesmith, 1985; Winkleman, 1994). Many students passed through the honeymoon phase and reached the crisis phase during the first week.

The crisis phase has been described as a period where "things start to go wrong, minor issues become major problems, and cultural differences become irritating" (Winkleman, 1994, p. 123). Students complained about the food choices, worried about sanitary conditions, and expressed feelings of suspiciousness and paranoia about being taken advantage of or cheated, robbed, or assaulted. Feelings of suspiciousness and paranoia were heightened by the minority status of the group (all female and Caucasian). Some students even found "innumerable reasons to dislike and criticize the culture" (Winkelman, 1994, p. 124).

To assist students to achieve the adjustment and reorientation phase, they are given an opportunity to express their feelings through group "post-conferences" with faculty at the end of each day. This approach to learning allows the students to focus on varying perceptions of reality and form a better understanding of the salient features of the phenomena they have experienced and problem-solve some of the difficulties they perceive. The need for these meetings diminishes with the length of stay, and overall, students come to appreciate the Jamaican culture and the challenges of negotiating in a foreign culture. Adaptation occurs in varying degrees from tolerance to fully embracing the culture.

Faculty serve in various capacities as they assist students through the phases of culture shock. Various roles identified by faculty at "Club Ed" include: teacher, clinician, mother-confessor, spiritual advisor, social worker, counselor, social director, tour guide, communications expert, insect control officer, ambassador, safety control officer, crisis intervention worker, and financier.

Role of the Faculty

Unlike traditional clinical experiences, nursing in the neighborhoods requires that the faculty give up any notion of direct supervision or control of the learning environment. Likewise, students need support in developing greater confidence in their abilities while, at the same time, recognizing the limits of their knowledge.

Faculty need to rely on their professional colleagues to assist in the teaching process. This requires that faculty dialogue these preceptors and assist them to understand and feel comfortable in their role in the process.

Role of the Community Providers

Students need encouragement to problem-solve and collaborate as a means of expanding their own knowledge. This collaboration includes sharing the process of teaching-learning and decision-making within the context of the student-client-preceptor interaction. To meet these objectives faculty role model critical thinking and learning as a life-long process. Students need to come to an understanding that it is not important to always have the answer, but it is important to be resourceful about finding answers (Shea, 1995, p. 35).

Agency staff and residents alike were encouraged to give feedback to students and faculty. Prior to working with the students, faculty met with the nurses and CHAs to discuss the students' objectives and the role that they would play in the process and to elicit their concerns. Unlike the agencies in which students have experiences in the U.S., this staff have had relatively little contact with students and welcome their presence. Some of the nurses expressed concerns about the students' abilities, but agency staff were reassured to know that students could only do what they (the student and preceptor) felt comfortable with doing.

Having the students in the clinic with their preceptors for a few days in advance of going out into the neighborhoods eased the preceptors' concerns. Preceptors were able to see the capabilities of the students and witness interactions between the faculty and students. This assisted the preceptors in understanding how faculty judge the readiness of a student for an experience.

Additionally, agency staff had minor concerns about malpractice issues in working with students, despite the fact that malpractice is not prevalent in the Jamaican health care system. Faculty offered agency staff reassurances that the students are covered under their own malpractice insurance and that the faculty are licensed as registered nurses in Jamaica. Though no formal mechanisms have been established, faculty make a point to check in with the agency staff on a daily basis to get a sense from them of how things are going. This gesture provides further opportunity for exchange. Additionally, faculty meet with the Senior Public Health Nurse to get indirect feedback. Overall, close communication is key to the success of this program. As we continue, more formalized means of evaluation are being developed between student, faculty, and preceptor.

Role of the Students

Students are responsible for meeting the needs of the residents in terms of culturally appropriate health care teaching, case finding, referrals, assessments, direct care, and follow-up home visits. Case-finding efforts are assisted by the nurse-midwives and CHAs who know of clients in need of well care, nutrition and developmental assessments, immunizations, or follow-up of individuals with chronic or acute diseases. An additional part of neighborhood rounds includes checking in on "shut-ins."

Role of the Residents

Residents of the neighborhood are actively encouraged to participate in the teaching-learning process. Clients are selected by the agency nurses and CHAs on the basis of continuity of care, services needed, and their availability and willingness to engage/participate with students. Students are encouraged to select a client-family on whom to center teaching-learning activities. Residents are encouraged to teach students about their cultural health needs, folkways, and practices. In interactions with staff and residents, the students are expected to conduct themselves in a culturally congruent manner. Students are assisted in this process by cultural immersion activities, the insights of staff and residents, and use of transcultural assessment tools.

While it is impossible for the faculty to meet with all of the residents with whom the students interacted, it is important from a relational perspective to know that student-resident interactions were going well. To the best of our abilities this is done through informal feedback mechanisms (putting our ears close to the ground) via agency staff, chance encounters with the families on return visits to the clinic, and neighborhood rounds with the driver where faculty "walked and talked about." This, at least, allows us the chance to demonstrate our concern for the welfare and needs of the residents participating in this process.

Formal mechanisms for evaluating the effectiveness of student-resident exchanges include student case studies, teaching projects, and journals. Once again, as the program continues to develop, methods are being developed to give the residents greater voice in the evaluative process.

ENVISIONING THE FUTURE

It is our hope that as we continue to return to these neighborhoods, the foundations that we have laid down will create greater opportunities for exchange. "To develop an educational partnership between the members of seemingly disparate settings, such as a college of nursing and a selected neighborhood, individuals of both locations need to work to develop a structure that enables all participants to interact and learn from each other" (Matteson, 1995, p. 55). This is the process that is evolving through a sharing of mutual expertise and understanding of each other's culture, subculture, norms, values, beliefs, customs, and folkways. We have gained entry and begun the process of relationship and trust-building. Returning faculty to the same neighborhoods for longitudinal experiences will be vital to the continuity necessary to assist in this process.

> *"It took a day or so for all of us to adjust to the clinic. After this, things started to move forward in terms of taking the initiative for and being able to do things. I performed postpartum exams, changed dressings, immunized infants, did nutritional counseling, family planning assessments and counseling. I've had some really amazing experiences here. In the community the learning opportunities were numerous . . . once I became accepted into a person's home I found it easier to ask questions, to see what would work in terms of treatments or teaching. I learned to ask for opportunities and to see opportunities in every experience"* (excerpt, Student Journal).

WHAT WE HAVE LEARNED

When embarking on such an experience, faculty need to recognize their own strengths and weaknesses, work together to balance each other, and be firmly aligned in what is communicated to students. This prevents unhealthy alliances from developing within the group. It is important to convey that there are multiple ways of viewing problems and that there is no one right way to learn. In addition, there must be a recognition and valuing of the strengths that the students bring to the experience and a valuing of them as persons. In hindsight, what was obscure now appears obvious. Faculty must enter this experience with an understanding that young adult learners, when severed from their usual coping mechanisms and resources, need to be assisted to find new ways of coping with the unfamiliar.

Faculty who engage in a program such as this need a keen sense of adventure and an interest in transcultural nursing as well as good critical thinking, problem solving, negotiation, and communication skills. In the clinical arena, a balance of interests and skills was also found to be help-ful in program planning and actualization of goals. In this case, the two faculty who attend represent a broad spectrum of family, maternal-child, and psychiatric-mental health specializations. This combination of clinical expertise has proved to be very helpful. Additionally, an important part of successful program planning was the familiarity of the course coordina-tor with the country and her expertise with regard to transcultural theory, Jamaican culture, and contacts within the country.

Throughout the trip the adventuresome group needs careful nurtur-ing. Faculty need to be emotionally present for the length of the program in order to ensure its success. Faculty may experience some of the same feelings of homesickness that the students experience. It is important as a part of group process to acknowledge these feelings, yet faculty need to maintain their role as leaders and deal with this in a thoughtful, mature manner that does not disrupt the group adaptation process. Anticipatory planning is required to ensure that a faculty member is able to manage cares with regard to home life at home. This is a crucial factor in the plan-ning process and requires careful consideration in the selection of indi-vidual faculty members. Other planning considerations include the ability of faculty to exist with little or no communication with the United States and their ability to adjust to the food and living accommodations. Faculty not only work closely but also often share accommodations, thus under-scoring the need for a balancing of strengths and weaknesses, a shared world view, and maturity in overlooking one another's peccadilloes.

In starting such an educational program, it is important to recognize at the outset that there is very little that is absolute and nearly everything is subject to change. Faculty must be willing to participate in a program where responsibility for the students is 24 hours-a-day, seven days-a-week for the duration of the assignment.

Faculty are responsible to the students in finding and creating the learning environment and then gaining the initial entry to the neighbor-hood (Matteson, 1995). This includes expressing to our colleagues the need for, and value of, a community-based and transcultural nursing experience within the existent nursing curriculum. Further, this required bargaining a role for ourselves and our students within the realm of the Jamaican health care organization. As we learned, successful negotiation through the front door does not necessarily guarantee full cooperation from all who interact with the students. "Maintaining a viable partnership within a relatively complex human organization is a continuous process and requires the efforts of all involved" (Matteson, 1995, p. 69).

In their infinite wisdom, faculty at DANE encouraged Hartwick faculty to become licensed as registered nurses in Jamaica as a means for negotiating better learning opportunities for students. This proved to be very helpful in those situations where preceptors had an initial reluctance to let students provide nursing care. In these situations faculty could assure the preceptor that the student could practice, according to agency regulations, under the faculty member's auspices. Once preceptors were able to see the student function autonomously, then they demonstrated a willingness to allow the students to practice "hands on."

Within each agency faculty spent time with the agency leaders, listening carefully to their needs and desires concerning the health of the community. Faculty worked with senior nurses within the clinics to arrange students' schedules. Time was spent explaining how the students might be able to assist with meeting one or several of their needs and helping staff to understand the ability levels of students.

Students were assisted by faculty in identifying potential learning situations and understanding how their abilities fit the situation. It was important to convey to the students that gaining trust is critical in terms of gaining access to the community and practice nursing care. This process required that students have patience, understanding, and a willingness to work within the norms and values of the system. Additionally, trust needed to evolve between the faculty and students, and students needed to be empowered as full partners in the teaching-learning process.

In planning a program, faculty need to start small and design realistic objectives. Course objectives should take into account what can be accomplished in a particular setting within the given time and cultural constraints. Objectives can be expanded as the relationship between academia and the neighborhood evolves. To enable growth of the program, it is vitally important that the faculty and students uphold the spirit and letter of any agreements. If faculty members and students fulfill their initial commitments, program expansion will come more readily (Matteson, 1995). Our welcome return to these settings is a testimonial to the time and energy that we have invested in this process of trust and mutual exchange.

Benefits to the Faculty

Despite the extent of planning involved, faculty benefit greatly from participation in such a program. First, it is gratifying to work in a collegial/collaborative relationship with faculty from another country. The development of this kind of relationship reaffirms what Leininger (1985) refers to as the universal as well as diverse meanings of nursing care. Second, faculty develop their own skills as culturally competent practitioners. Third, students and faculty have the chance to develop different relationships that allow each a better understanding of the others as persons and professionals. Fourth, faculty learn to let go of preconceived notions that only nurses can teach nursing and learn that educational opportunities present themselves in a variety of settings—including the beach—if one is open to them. Finally, faculty may benefit positively from an understanding that students seek self-actualization as learners, are often aware of what they need to learn, and, if given the chance, will look for these opportunities.

One of the many joys of the days in Jamaica was the ambiance created by using the natural backdrop of the beach for post-conferences. These student-faculty interactions often occurred by candlelight after dark. This setting freed students to share thoughts and feelings that were controversial, unacceptable, and/or challenging. The soothing sounds of the ocean and the soft candlelight minimized distractions and allowed the students to open up to one another.

Benefits to Students

Students self-selected into the program based on their own interests and an understanding of their own learning needs. Important considerations included future career goals consistent with international or community nursing, a desire to work in urban centers where large, multicultural populations seek health care, or an interest in transcultural nursing theory. Currently the ability to finance the trip weighs heavily into this decision-making process, however, sources of outside funding are being sought to eliminate this possible bias.

Students who self-select into this program are, by virtue of this process, risk-takers. Ideally, students who engage in such a program need to be flexible and creative. Certainly, students need to be successful academically in meeting course prerequisites. In larger schools of nursing, a more refined selection process would be imperative, and this might include an interview process, an essay on career objectives or the like. In a small program such as ours, students are well-known to faculty so the process in much less formal.

Prior to embarking on this journey students are expected to attend a series of meetings in which various aspects of the trip are addressed. Discussions center around diet, customs, bartering, history of the country, and health care issues. Practical aspects of the trip are discussed including the travel itinerary, accommodations, eating arrangements, means of communication, and packing instructions. Students are all required to have proof of appropriate immunizations, a WHO health card, and a U.S. passport or other appropriate identification. Sanitary issues are reviewed and students are urged to bring prophylactic medications and re-hydration supplies in the event of traveler's diarrhea. Additionally, students are encouraged to carry with them any prescription medications that they anticipate they might need for routine illnesses.

Course preparation includes a reading list of scholarly journal articles and popular literature to give students some idea of the culture and experience they will be encountering. Course packets of copyrighted materials were developed through library services. Suggestions for the reading list come from various faculty who have had transcultural experiences in Jamaica or the Caribbean as well as from our Caribbean colleagues at the DANE. According to Bartol (1989), reading literature allows one to live an experience vicariously. Viewed from afar, the material is less threatening and provides a basis for understanding a culture (Bartol & Richardson, 1998).

Upon arrival in Jamaica, the orientation becomes a 24 hour-a-day, seven day-a-week process. Students are informally oriented to their surroundings by drivers, walking tours of the neighborhoods, and facilities with DANE faculty and agency staff. The orientation continues through attendance at local church services, interactions at local stores, and with local vendors and community members. Students and faculty alike need to be constantly aware of their inherent ambassadorial role.

"I knew that my actions would not only reflect on who I was, but also my group, Hartwick College, even the U.S." (excerpt, Student Journal)

Through ongoing discussions, students are assisted to see themselves in the context of the "bigger picture" as ambassadors for the college, the profession, and their country. In light of these responsibilities, it is impressed upon students, prior to disembarking and throughout the trip, the need to maintain good public relations and present themselves in a manner consistent with acceptable cultural norms. Professionally, students are encouraged to provide culturally competent care.

In terms of collegial relationships, students are assisted to be sensitive to the power differentials inherent in student-staff relationships, particularly in the context of a foreign educational system. In the Jamaican system of education, greater deference is shown to one's teachers and being overly familiar without invitation to do so might be construed as disre-spectful. Students are encouraged to address their preceptors in the cus-tomary Jamaican fashion as "Nurse. . . ."

Additionally, students are encouraged to be open-minded and reserve judgment with respect to the health care system and customs of the Jamaican. What students discover is that, as outsiders, it is easy to judge harshly, but as one gets to know and understand the people, the culture, and the system, respect for their accomplishments in light of priority set-ting and limited resources grows.

> *"At times I wish I could have put my two cents in or changed something I was seeing, but I realize that that is a reflection of my own values. I came here with a set of values that have continuously been called into question. I have seen many things that have made me appreciate what I have, and I have come to appreciate other things as well."* (excerpt, Student Journal)

One interesting insight gained by students was an understanding of the importance of education to change, not unlike what Gmelch's students found in Barbados (1994). Hartwick students meet Jamaican students who view education as a privilege versus a right. The Hartwick nursing stu-dents learn a new appreciation of their relative ease to access education when in a country where students compete for limited spaces in the class-room and work hard to earn the money and gain the privilege to take entrance exams for high school and college. As students in a university program, Hartwick nursing students are accorded respect by those with whom they interact.

Often through a process of trial and error, students discover the cul-tural relativity of what is "politically correct" in terms of human interac-tions. As a group of female students, they learn about the directness of the young Jamaican male and, under the good-humored tutelage of some young Jamaican women, how to handle unwanted advances in an equally direct yet respectful manner. Peer interactions are an important part of the education process.

Students assist in the neighborhoods and community-based clinics on a case-by-case basis. What takes place in the nurse-client encounter depends upon how the situation presents itself, the priorities involved, and the resources and capabilities of the individual client, student, and health care system. Aside from typical clinic and home visit encounters, students are invited to speak to groups of clients in waiting rooms at pre-natal, family planning, and well-child clinics on any number of subjects. Opportunities for teaching also arise at local schools and an orphanage. Each of these opportunities presents an opportunity for the students to give back to a community that is so generously investing time and energy in their educational experience.

When traveling in a country with limited financial, material, and human resources, students are challenged to provide care in a resourceful manner. Use of limited resources requires prioritization, critical thinking, and ingenuity. Additionally, being in a different culture requires an understanding of the need to incorporate strategies that are congruent with the person's beliefs and capabilities. Students quickly learn the need to provide culturally congruent care. They discover the importance of incorporating traditional, homeopathic, and spiritual beliefs into the plan of care while still promoting the health of persons.

One particular student was challenged when working with a Rastafarian family of a young asthmatic who was, in concert with his spiritual beliefs, smoking ganja (marijuana). Through exploration of the health-related effects of smoking and the meaning of ganja in the context of the client's physical health, it was agreed that the client could still meet his spiritual needs without exacerbating his health problems by making ganja infusions (teas).

Students working in the day care center were similarly challenged when they witnessed corporal punishment practices that ran counter to their own beliefs about disciplining children. Initially, students felt powerless in terms of making a difference, but through careful exploration of the ideology that gives rise to this form of discipline, students began to understand their ability to function as role models in demonstrating alternative approaches. Students were encouraged to begin this process by engaging in discussions with teachers and parents about discipline. This experience assisted students to understand the cultural relativity of norms and sanctions, the need to tread lightly and not judge too harshly less they loose any opportunity that they might have to introduce change.

Students are encouraged to share their learning experiences through reflective post-conferencing and journal writing. These mechanisms allow faculty to keep in touch with what the students are experiencing, assist the students in processing these experiences and promote adaptation and learning. Additional teaching-learning experiences include presentation of case studies. In the future, these case studies may serve as a further means of sharing with our international colleagues.

Establishing a Longitudinal Experience

While students do "rotate" to different areas within the clinic (i.e., medical clinic, dressing clinic, prenatal clinic, etc.), they are able to establish continuity through their community health preceptors and clients. Students are encouraged to establish connections with families in the neighborhoods and follow those families as they interacted with the health care system. Generally, home visits are made twice weekly. The preceptors are key in providing students with insights into the needs of the families and formalizing the linkages between the students and families. At the end of the experience, termination is eased by the knowledge that continuity will be maintained by the preceptor.

In one case, the student and her preceptor worked with the breast-feeding mother of an infant that was "failing to thrive." The infant was being followed because the infant's weight at four months of age was equivalent to its birth weight. During a home visit, the student assessed that the infant was well below the developmental milestones for weight and longitudinal growth. The student discussed her concerns with the mother. The mother related that she had breastfed her other children and they had not experienced any problems with weight gain. The mother, however, was feeding this infant weakened tea because she was refusing to suckle at the breast for more than a few minutes at a time.

The student, in collaboration with the mother and the CHA, referred the infant to the clinic for a nurse check and nutrition referral. The next day, the student was pleased to see that the mother brought the infant to the clinic. The student accompanied the mother when she went to see the nurse-midwife. It was discovered that the infant had a bad case of thrush. The student went with the mother to the pharmacist to obtain the medication and then provided the mother with instructions on how to use the medication as well as other measures that would help eradicate the yeast infection.

The student continued to follow this mother-infant dyad and her family in the home. The infant began gaining weight, the mother returned to the clinic for both family planning and nutritional counseling, and she brought the infant in to update her immunizations. These events all transpired in a couple weeks, and while there were no additional problems, when the students left the case was turned over to the CHA for continued monitoring.

Clearly, this case demonstrates how nursing in the neighborhoods functions to benefit the people by developing liaisons between the members of the community and the agency. In addition, there are indirect benefits to the agency staff when students provide care. It allows agency staff time to work on indirect patient care-planning, scheduling, restocking, quality assurance, and administrative activities. Students and faculty also bring gifts of time, energy, equipment, supplies, and knowledge in exchange for the numerous learning opportunities proffered.

An indirect benefit to the neighborhood is the boost to the local economy provided by students' buying meals everyday, utilizing local transportation providers, and supporting local church programs. Less tangible but certainly of importance is the opportunity for the members of the community to meet non-tourists from the United States and be exposed to different ideas, lifestyles, customs, values, and beliefs.

Reflecting on Culture

Through journal entries that included narrative and critical analysis, students identify personal values and beliefs that impact on interactions with and care of persons of a different culture. Not unlike themes identified by Gmelch (1992, 1994), students reflect on their feelings about being members of a minority, the subtle as well as stark differences in social class, and the interdependent and intimate nature of community life as it contrasts with the impersonal, autonomous and detached life they experience at home. Journals reflect a struggle to adjust to the cultural relativity of time as evidenced in the statement, "Soon Come." Additionally, within groups of students some have more difficulty adjusting to changes in diet, accommodations, and the absence of diversional activities and instant entertainment readily available at home. The majority of students adjust and come to realize how privileged they have been to see "the real Jamaica." Many students state that they are struck by how little most tourists know about Jamaica and the arrogance of the tourist lifestyle. Many students also comment on the contentment of the Jamaican people despite their lack of material goods and the centrality of their religious beliefs to their happiness.

Hopefully, with continued reflection students will gain, as Gmelch (1992) found:

> ". . . a more critical perspective on their own culture—its materialism, conspicuous consumption, and not always benign influence on the developing world. They became more respectful of other cultures, having learned that their own culture doesn't always have all the answers and that other values and perspectives are equally worthy and, in fact, sometimes make more sense." (p. 250)

Understanding Others

Traditional (Tylerian) curricular models in nursing education emphasize behavioral objectives, outcomes, products, and a priori content. State Boards of Nursing and accrediting agencies have encouraged educators to embrace this behavioral paradigm. While the Tylerian model has led to some important contributions to nursing, its dominance in nursing education has created serious concerns related to students' abilities to know and understand the cultural meanings of health, illness, healing, care, and caring. It has also limited critical and creative thinking about world-wide cultural realities (Andrews, 1995).

Students need educational opportunities that: assist them in seeing cultural similarities and differences between and among cultural groups/individuals; emphasize universal human phenomena and requisites; and assist them to see themselves and others as members of the human race. These opportunities will assist them in identifying potential strengths and limitations in their knowledge and/or skill in providing culturally competent care, foster their interaction with clients representing various cultures and subcultures, and enable them to apply transcultural principles, concepts, theories, and research findings as a foundation to practice. All nursing care is transcultural (Andrews, 1995).

SUMMARY

Nursing in the neighborhoods in Jamaica has offered students and faculty a unique experience to focus on the meanings, values, and practices of care within this specific cultural and community context. Through this experience, students have been assisted to "discover and explain ways that culturally constituted care contributes to the health and well being of people" (Leininger, 1995, 1997, p. 342). This professional competence must be seen as encompassing cultural competence and become an integral part of ". . . preparing a competent, humanistic, practitioner" (AAN, 1995, p. 16).

The program abroad engages the students in a 24 hour-a-day, seven day-a-week cultural immersion experience in the community creating a greater than what occurs in hospital-based setting where students are exposed on a limited basis to persons of a different culture. This concentrated learning experience helps students to understand the "lived experience" of a people.

Engaging in such an experience may limit students' exposure to the high technology interventions and sophisticated treatments available in modern Western health care institutions. This is counterbalanced, however, by the ability to engage in opportunities that foster cultural competence where "the importance of dialogue, meaning, self-reflection, intuition, and praxis" (Andrews, 1995, p. 5) are employed.

REFERENCES

Adler, P. (1975). *The transitional experience: An alternative view of cultural shock. Journal of Humanistic Psychology, 15,* 183–204.

American Academy of Nursing. (1995). *Promoting cultural competence in and through nursing education.* Washington, D.C.: Author.

American Association of Colleges of Nursing. (1998). *The essentials of baccalaureate education for professional nursing practice.* Washington, DC: AACN.

American Nurse's Association. (1991). *Standards of clinical nursing practice.* Washington, D.C.: Author.

Andrews, M. (1995). *Transcultural Nursing: Transforming the curriculum. Journal of Transcultural Nursing, 6*(2), 4–9.

Baker, C. P. (1996). *Jamaica: A lonely plant travel survival kit.* Hawthorne, Australia: Lonely Planet Publications.

Bartol, G. M. (1989). *Creative literature: An aid to nursing practice. Nursing and Health Care, 10,* 453–457.

Bartol, G. M. & Richardson, L. (1998). *Using literature to create cultural competence. Image: Journal of Nursing Scholarship, 30*(1), 75–79.

Campinha-Bacote, J., Yahle, T. & Langenkamp, M. (1998). *The challenge of cultural diversity for nurse educators.* In J. Campinha-Bacote. (1998). *Readings and resources in transcultural health care and mental health,* 10th ed., 121–135.

Catlin, A. (1996). *Interview and observations: Nurse Practitioners in Jamaica. Image: Journal of Nursing Scholarship, 28*(4), 370.

Clinton, J. F. (1996). *Cultural diversity and health care in America: Knowledge fundamental to cultural competence in baccalaureate nursing students, Journal of Cultural Diversity, 3*(3), 4–8.

Degazon, C. E. & Fieldo, S. B. (1997). *When cultures collide. Nursing and Health Care Perspectives, 18*(5), 238–243.

Fletcher, V. C. (1997). *Where is nursing's role in promoting culturally competent care? Lifelines, 6,* p. 13.

Frei, F., Hugentobler, M., Schurman, S., Duell, W. & Alioth, A. (1994). *Work design for the competent organization.* Westport, CT: Quorom Books.

Furnham, A. & Bochner, S. (1986). *Culture shock.* London: Methuen.

Gmelch, G. (1992). *Learning culture: The education of American students in Caribbean villages. Human Organization, 51*(3), 245–251.

Gmelch, G. (1994). *Lessons from the field.* In J. P. Spradley and D. W. McCurdy, (1994). *Conformity & Conflict,* 8th ed., 45–55.

Hart, K. (1989). *Women and the sexual division of labour in the Caribbean.* Kingston: The Consortium graduate School of Social Sciences.

Hartwick College. (1998). *Hartwick College Catalog, 1998–2000.* New York: Hartwick College.

Kulwicki, A. & Boloink, B. J. (1996). *Assessment of level of comfort in providing multi-cultural nursing care by baccalaureate nursing students. Journal of Cultural Diversity, 3*(2), 40–45.

Leavitt, R. L. (1992). *Disability and rehabilitation in rural Jamaica: An ethnographic study.* Rutherford: Farleigh Dickinson University Press.

Leininger, M. (1985). *Transcultural care diversity and universality: A theory of nursing. Nursing and Health Care, 64*(4), 209–212.

Leninger, M. (1995). *Nursing theories and culture: Fit or misfit? Journal of Transcultural Nursing, 7*(1), 41–42.

Leninger, M. (1997). *Transcultural nursing research to transform nursing education and practice: 40 years. Image: Journal of Nursing Scholarship, 29*(4), 341–347.

Logan, J. R. (1995). *Rural America as a symbol of American values. Rural development perspectives, 12*(1), pp. 24–28.

Matteson, P. S. (Ed.). (1995). *Teaching nursing in the neighborhoods: The Northeastern model*. New York: Springer.

Momsen, J. H. (1993). *Women and Change in the Caribbean*. Kingston: Ian Randle.

National League for Nursing (1993). *A vision for nursing education*. New York: Author.

Newman, M. A. (1986). *Health as expanding consciousness*. St. Louis: Mosby.

Orlandi, M. A. (Ed.) (1992). *Cultural competence for evaluators*. Washington, D.C.: Department of Health and Human Services.

Rhinesmith, S. (1985). *Bringing home the new world*. New York: Walsh.

Shea, C. A. (1995). *Laying the groundwork for curriculum change*. In P. S. Matteson (Ed.). *Teaching nursing in the neighborhoods: The Northeastern model*. New York: Springer.

Spitzer, A., Kesselring, A., Ravid, C., Tamir, B., Granot, M., and Noam, R. (1996). *Learning about another culture: Project and curricular reflections. Journal of Nursing Education, 35*(7), 3222–328.

Winkleman, M. (1994). *Cultural shock and adaptation. Journal of Counseling and Development, 73*(2), 121–133.

Wuest, J. (1992). Joining together: Students and faculty learn about transcultural nursing. *Journal of Nursing Education, 31*(2), 90–92.

9

The Vision on 22nd Street Partnership: The Experience of Cleveland State University (Ohio)

Cheryl P. McCann and Sheila A. Niles

The stimulus to develop a community-based curriculum at Cleveland State University in the Department of Nursing resulted from three events that converged and provided a framework for the paradigm shift. Two events were external to the department and one was internal and faculty-generated.

The more general factors that captured our interest were the recommendations from the Pew Health Professions Commission (PEW), the American Academy of Colleges of Nursing (AACN), and the National League for Nursing (NLN) that nursing education was to encompass more community-based nursing education. Within the previous decade, a national trend in health care delivery had shifted away from the acute care setting to community-based service delivery models. Observing this trend, Pew, AACN, and the NLN recommended that nursing education develop new models of integration between education and practice. These models would provide nursing students with education and clinical practice that they would need to provide care within the nation's changing health care system.

More locally, a partnership/alliance was formed between the Department of Nursing at Cleveland State University and the Visiting Nurses Association of Cleveland. The partnership occurred when the strategic plans of two institutions, Cleveland State University (CSU) and the Visiting Nurse Association of Cleveland (VNA), representing education and service, identified "shared needs" and the "added values" that would be achieved through this unique alliance. In 1993, the President and Board of Trustees of CSU and the President/CEO and Board of Trustees of the VNA committed human, fiscal, and material resources to initiate the multifaceted process that resulted in a fully integrated, community-based model know as Vision on 22nd Street. By restructuring the CSU nursing curriculum and the VNA practice setting, a seamless process was formed to prepare undergraduate nursing students for community-based practice. The successful development of the partnership was facilitated by the shared values, needs, and missions of each organization as well as their geographic proximity, 22nd Street.

Internally, some faculty within the Department of Nursing had already considered the idea of this paradigm shift. In the early 1990s, in response to national trends in the location of heath care sites, faculty in some clinical courses began providing a variety of experiential community-based learning activities for students in nursing specialty courses. The most pronounced changes were in the area of behavioral health, sometimes identified as mental health, which was rapidly shifting from institutional to community-based treatment. Since the theoretical framework of the curriculum emphasized a health promotion-disease prevention model, this shift in clinical education sites in a course fit well. It then provided a bridge to developing a community-based curriculum and a creative response to the national trends in health care delivery.

PARTNERS IN EDUCATION
CLEVELAND STATE UNIVERSITY

Cleveland State University is an urban university located in downtown Cleveland, Ohio. CSU students reflect the diversity of the Cleveland urban and suburban populations. The goals and mission of the CSU Department of Nursing, one of 24 programs housed within the College of Arts and Science, mirror those of the university. One goal in particular is to analyze and selectively strengthen partnerships. The department has chosen to "engage in partnerships with community agencies to implement the goals of the curriculum and to enhance the public's health."

Currently there are 11 full-time faculty, four who are tenured. The student population (n=200) includes a Registered Nurse to Bachelor of Science in Nursing (RN-BSN) track which has been in existence for 20 years and a basic Bachelor of Science in Nursing (BSN) track that was initiated in 1997.

Approximately half of the students within the nursing major reside in the urban area around the university. The other half are split between the eastern and the western suburbs. At least 10% of each class is male, with minority representation that includes Americans of African, Middle Eastern, Asian, Hispanic, and Russian descent. Approximately 85% of the graduates will remain in the area. Approximately one-third of the BSN nursing students and over half of the RN-BSN graduates pursue graduate education.

Reflecting the diversity of an urban population the nursing classes are often evenly divided between traditional college age students and non-traditional college students. Clinical experiences are obtained for students learning throughout the Greater Cleveland area with affiliations in more than 30 health-related settings.

PARTNERS IN EDUCATION VISITING NURSES ASSOCIATION OF CLEVELAND

Founded in 1902, the Visiting Nurse Association of Cleveland is the oldest voluntary community health organization in Ohio. Its mission is to provide innovative, cost effective, high-quality health care to all people by delivering services to promote health, independence, and dignity; to teach people to care for themselves and each other; and to provide additional services to the poor as VNA funds permit.

The VNA offers a comprehensive range of skilled home care services, disease management programs, and health promotion and wellness programs to the eight counties of the Greater Cleveland community. Services include skilled nursing care, elder care, occupational and physical therapy, infusion therapy, mental health services, hospice care, pediatric and maternal health care, home health aide and homemaker services, HIV/AIDs care, and social work services.

The VNA is accredited with the Joint Commission of Accreditation of Health Care Organizations (JCAHO). It is governed by a community Board of Trustees and its committees including a Professional Advisory Committee, a Research Advisory Committee, and an Ethics Advisory Committee. Its long history of providing community health care, offering skills in health promotion and disease prevention, and providing referrals and linkages to existing community resources while remaining an independent agency demonstrates its expertise and service value to the community.

THE NEIGHBORHOOD

Both organizations are located on 22nd Street in downtown Cleveland, Ohio. The areas surrounding and served by these institutions are multicultural, impoverished, and heavily populated within a relatively small geographic area. Housing projects and business areas stand side by side. Numerous health care facilities are within blocks of one another, including community hospitals and the health care giants, Cleveland Clinic Foundation and the University Hospitals of Cleveland.

THE CURRICULUM OF NEIGHBORHOOD-BASED NURSING EDUCATION

The Vision on 22nd Street model was conceptualized as an education/ practice model to restructure nursing education within this institution. The process of development of the model brought together nurse experts from divergent areas of practice, academia, and service. The members of the VNA and the CSU faculty were equal partners in the development process. Ongoing discussions created group consensus around the modifications that needed to be made in order to reflect the beliefs and ideas of both groups. Together they created the Vision on 22nd Street mission statement, established goals, and determined the curricular and practice components of this community-based curriculum.

The Vision's theoretical framework, building on the stress models of Selye and Antonovsky (1976, 1979), encompasses concepts of health promotion and disease prevention within the context of stress and adaptation. Major concepts include communication, critical thinking, research, use of the nursing process, the multiple roles of the nurse, and the ethical and legal considerations of practice. The curriculum is structured so that concepts are presented from simple to complex, tertiary prevention to primary prevention, and individual to family, group, and community as client.

Faculty believe that baccalaureate education should produce an educated person who has command of the cognitive, psychomotor, and affective domains of learning. Clinical experiences are an integral component of the overall plan of study, with each didactic course having an accompanying clinical component. With this nursing education program, community-based concepts and experiential activities now are a part of every classroom and clinical course.

When the curriculum was revised to incorporate community as a major curricular concept, a curriculum grid was constructed which detailed the major concepts incorporated into each classroom and clinical course, the teaching learning strategies, the community concepts, and the community-based activities.

Concepts within courses are grounded within the level of prevention upon which the course is framed (primary, secondary, or tertiary) and is concept-specific for a given specialty area (adult health, maternal-child health, behavioral health, or community). Students are introduced to clinical practice beginning in the first semester of the sophomore year. The sophomore year courses concentrate on tertiary preventive strategies such as chronic illness and aging. The junior year focuses on secondary preventive strategies such as acute care of adults and the specialty focuses of care. The senior courses emphasize primary prevention.

With each subsequent clinical course students are expected to successfully demonstrate their ability to perform specific psychomotor skills within a laboratory prior to practice in the clinical arena. Psychomotor skills and knowledge of underlying rationale progress in degree of sophistication as the student progresses from sophomore to senior. As an example, medication administration progresses from oral medication to intramuscular and intravenous administration. After demonstrating preparation of a sterile field, the student learns application of a sterile dressing, wound irrigation and packing, catheterization, etc. While the goal of the faculty working in the courses is to present didactic content at the same time students are learning laboratory skills, time parameters with a course do not always allow the teaching and the practice to be evenly matched.

Clinical practice assignments always assume the ability of the student to execute specific psychomotor skills, having done so first in a simulated setting. Additional expectations in each clinical course include selected community-based experiential activities, the ability to critically think and problem-solve, and safe performance of required nursing care in the assigned environments.

CONNECTING WITH THE NEIGHBORHOODS

Cleveland's inner-city neighborhoods are rich in culturally diverse ethnic populations. The 22nd Street Partnership reaches out to these neighborhoods through the Neighborhood Centers Association (NCA). This Association is comprised of 23 autonomous social service agencies that provide emergency services (i.e., food, shelter, clothing) for the poor and for homeless people, day care for children and older adults, residential care, and congregate meal sites (nutrition services) for older adults. These agencies operate independently in the settlement house tradition, work with established community boards, and have served the Cleveland community since the early 1900s. Learning the needs of the residents is accomplished through neighborhood focus groups combined with knowledge gained through community-based faculty practice.

NEIGHBORHOOD-BASED EDUCATION

In collaboration with neighborhood centers and, in some instances, with the VNA providing entrée, CSU has established clinical activities in sites where structured programs are already in place, such as a program called Healthy Town.

Healthy Town: Neighborhood Health Connection

In 1994, the VNA of Cleveland responded to the health care needs articulated in focus groups with the executive directors of the agencies of the NCA. In response to and in collaboration with the target neighborhoods, the VNA initiated a grant-funded program labeled Healthy Town: Neighborhood Health Connection. This Healthy Town initiative provides health promotion and disease prevention services to low-income inner-city residents. The goals of Healthy Town are: 1) to provide health promotion and disease prevention services that improve the clients' health states; 2) to provide health promotion and disease prevention training to staff, volunteers, and outreach workers at the target neighborhood centers where services are delivered; and 3) to refer and link clients to existing health care and community resources.

The Healthy Town initiative provides the CSU Department of Nursing with opportunities to expand the scope of clinical sites for undergraduate community-based care. As a result of this multifaceted collaboration, the Healthy Town grant funding has been sustained and the projects continue, with the CSU faculty as students as integral participants.

During the past three years, one of the most successful health promotion and disease prevention activities has been providing flu immunizations to home-bound elderly, with case finding through the community centers. In 1998, over 300 immunizations were given. A protocol was developed for student assessment of these home-bound elders to evaluate or gauge their need for additional services. This activity demonstrates the collaboration that occurs between neighborhood centers, city health departments, and the Healthy Town program of the VNA.

One Healthy Town neighborhood site with a diverse population has a number of specific programs in place. They have welcomed the students with open arms. The site provides a hunger center, a senior center, day care programs for children and for seniors, and a half-way house and group homes nearby. Students have become data collectors for a grant secured by the center director. They assess the pediatric health and developmental levels of the children while observing them in after-school activities.

ROLE OF THE PROVIDERS IN THE NEIGHBORHOODS

University and neighborhood social service contracts with clearly delineated expectations have been developed for all clinical sites. In nearly all instances, the neighborhood sites requested the following information about the nursing students coming to them: validation of current immunizations, malpractice insurance, and an assurance of the student's health. Recently, some have requested validation of student health insurance. Agency concerns about the screening of students being placed with them reflect an increased awareness of self-advocacy at the grass roots level in the neighborhood.

Providers in the neighborhood meet with the faculty responsible for the course prior to the student's arrival. At that time, they share a syllabus, course expectations, and guide sheets or written requirements that students will have. They also share their ideas about projects, plans, and programming where they would welcome students input and participation.

Providers have input into the evaluation process, providing information about student performance, freely sharing both accolades and concerns. The faculty, however, are ultimately responsible for assigning a clinical grade (all of our clinical courses have a letter grade).

Responses from providers about the students have been overwhelmingly positive. For example, in one setting the director includes student activities in her yearly plans for health teaching, work with seniors and children, and new programs planning. At the present time, one senior is completing her practicum at the center. One project involves implementing an intergenerational fair with plans that will later culminate in an ongoing intergenerational program.

Another student who recently worked with seniors at the center won a prize for a poster submitted to reflect activities of students in the community. This student presented the check received to further develop already existing programming efforts for seniors and matched the check with his own funds.

FACULTY INVOLVEMENT IN THE NEIGHBORHOODS

An evolving community-based curriculum presents challenges in faculty assignment within the neighborhoods. Critical to successful assignment of faculty to community-based activities are expertise in community practice, workload, and a committed interest in the work.

All 11 faculty members in the Department of Nursing participated in the development of Vision on 22nd Street. Enthusiasm for the model varied, however, in part because all participation had to be accomplished in addition to each faculty member's regular workload. Only two faculty members had experience working with the community. Others, familiar with institutional settings such as critical care, have been skeptical that community clinical experiences will adequately prepare students for the reality of the workplace.

Through faculty practice, two faculty continue to collaborate with the neighborhoods, meeting their evolving neighborhood needs. One faculty member developed an opportunity for students to provide the assessment and screening of children in a neighborhood day care center. They evaluate their health status, identify developmental delays, and make the necessary referrals. A second faculty member has created a program of screening elders for health care and other needs and then matching the community resources available in lieu of nursing home placements. These faculty practices provide role modeling for students and communicate the reality of allocation of resources and services in the community.

Faculty with responsibilities for student experiences in the neighborhoods develop strategies that allow students to provide care safety within the neighborhood. For instance, in the behavioral health course, some students visit clients in pairs. In addition, student activities are scheduled during the day, with assignments and time frames well-known to the faculty.

Faculty are provided with beepers, and most faculty have a personal cellular phone. With full implementation of the Vision on 22nd Street educational model and ongoing student participation, however, anxiety appears to be decreasing. Students have expressed less fear of being in the community through both self-report and the evaluation of their experiences. Perhaps learning the didactic concept of community as an environment of care coupled with the simultaneous entry into the neighborhoods in the sophomore year results in a more confident student, more understanding of clients' lives, and better prepared to deal with providing care within neighborhood situations.

Students within the nursing major have multiple opportunities to experience one or more of the Cleveland neighborhoods. Students are able, based upon the number of credit hours earned, to choose their clinical sites. Registration for a specific site is dependent upon student status, with seniors having priority.

Some choose to experience a number of different sites while others prefer to stay in one geographic area throughout their major. While the Vision partnership has afforded opportunities for students to experience urban Cleveland neighborhoods, others select clinical experiences in suburbia.

ORIENTATION OF STUDENTS TO THE NEIGHBORHOOD

The concept of the community as an environment of care is first introduced during the orientation to the nursing major. Issues such as safety, appropriate professional behavior, and the use of interpersonal skills are incorporated into discussions in all courses. The Vision partnership provides opportunities for students and university faculty to participate in the ongoing components of VNA's safety and training inservices educational programs. With student classrooms in the VNA building, participants are able to interact in both the formal and informal educational sessions with the staff on a daily basis.

Students are oriented to their assigned neighborhood on the first clinical day. Orientation varies dependent upon the neighborhood chosen by the student and the expectations for the student experience. The bulk of the orientation may fall upon the person with whom the student is working in a particular site, although faculty always carry out a portion of the orientation as well. Without exception, faculty meet with the students and discuss course expectations prior to any entry into a community site. At that time they also address situations and issues about which students should be cognizant.

In the behavioral health (mental health) course, students are placed in a setting (crisis shelter, halfway house, city mission, and group home) generally in pairs, but sometimes independently. In these situations, the faculty member has determined which students will be placed in a specific site. The faculty initially prepare the student with information about the site and then the provider continues the orientation. The provider actively participates in the evaluation process by meeting (or speaking with) the faculty periodically throughout the student's experience.

Two basic students in this course were so impressed with the work done within their site that, following the course, they returned to present a series of continuing education programs for the participants. A student in another site (a half way house), in collaboration with the staff, treated the occupants to dinner and a movie following her clinical course completion. These students are not only connecting with the clients with their heads but also their hearts.

In some clinical courses during the senior year, students are assigned to a home care agency for skilled home care services, and to a community center. Within the semester, students are then able to view the community from different parameters and perspectives.

RESULTS OF THE NEIGHBORHOOD PARTNERSHIP

Students

Anecdotal data and faculty observation has determined that, as a result of participation in this program, most students see community as a credible practice environment and one where nursing must be developed in order to provide competent care. They see the community as a setting they would consider for practice. Many students still express that their problem-solving and technical skills must be honed for a year following graduation before they embark upon a position in the community. The source of this belief has not yet been determined. One basic student who is a community-oriented, adult learner approached a faculty member just prior to graduation to let her know that community was the practice setting of choice, but expressed concern that, as a new graduate, the ability to problem-solve may not be firmly enough developed. Benner's perceptions about the development of a nurse were discussed and the act of maturing over time, no matter what the setting (1984). With that reassurance, the student is interviewing for a position offered through the VNA to our graduates.

The curriculum and its experiences have heightened cultural sensitivity in a way that reading about and discussing such issues can never match. Faculty report that the community experiences have influenced the way in which students provide care as evidenced by entries in their care plans, discussions in their critical thought journals, and the information they present when teaching their clients. They also appear to have a better understanding about the illness experience across settings.

Neighborhood Partners

One goal of the Vision partnership has been that graduates are knowledgeable about and ready to practice in the community. More specifically, the activities have resulted in improved coordination of health education services to targeted neighborhoods. While longitudinal data collection determines the extent of the progress toward that goal, we do know that many previously unmet neighborhood needs have been fulfilled since the beginning of the partnership.

For example:

- Partnership collaboration supported Healthy Town funding with CSU faculty and students as integral to the continuation of the projects in the neighborhoods.

- Increased flu immunizations for home-bound elders (N=300).
- Assessment of health needs to home-bound elders served by neighborhood center home delivered meals (N=300).
- Increased educational programs and inservices based upon neighborhood needs, i.e., infection control, hand washing, diabetic foot care, nutrition classes, health fairs (N=178).
- Assessment of developmental delays for selected day care center children (N=40).
- Skilled home care visits by the RN to BSN students (N=172) and the basic nursing students (N=300).
- Mental or behavioral health visits (N=400).
- Service to group homes such as education and environmental assessments for community students and for behavioral health students (N=120).
- Support visits to assisted living residents such as environmental, physical, and psychomotor assessment (N=100).
- Effective discharge planning and coordination of community resources.
- Improved coordination of health care services, i.e., research.
- Improved coordination of health education services to selected neighborhoods.

For the Faculty

Maintaining ongoing interest for faculty not originally developed within the Vision model has been problematic at times, mainly because of faculty turnover in both the academic and service arenas. This turnover has not been related to the project but to issues such as moving, better paying job in the service sector, promotions with new job, and tenure and promotion issues. The result has been the need for ongoing faculty development and bringing new faculty on board. A self-study and NLN re-accreditation, a university switch from quarters to semesters, and the search for a new department chair have further complicated the process. These diversions are now at an end. Those faculty who were initially part of joint faculty development continue to buy in and express support for the project. Many continually look to find additional ways to enhance community experiences which already exist through modifications in lectures and the never-ending search for community-inclusive texts.

One goal of the Vision model was to build a learning community through research, education, and practice. One approach to fulfilling that goal is CSU faculty practice at the VNA during the summer. This year, two faculty are employed within the agency during the summer months. Not only are they becoming more knowledgeable about the neighborhoods and the community resources, but they are also gaining expertise that they will be able to share with students regarding the community and its needs. They will also be able to share with students the complex information technology systems that are used for documentation within the VNA system.

Faculty in community, behavioral health, and some of the medical/surgical courses continue to refine lectures and explore textbooks with applications to community. Those faculty who continue to have the most difficulty integrating concepts of community-based care are the medical-surgical faculty. Most have never been exposed to community (except during their BSN program), and their nursing careers have centered around the high-tech world of the hospital. One clinical faculty member practicing as a part-time staff nurse this summer at the VNA is a critical care nurse. She explained that she appreciates the complexities of home care and wants to better understand the issues involved for clients when they leave the acute care environment.

DETERRENTS TO IMPLEMENTATION OF PROGRAM

A major barrier was the time commitment needed to develop and implement the project. Based upon a time line developed in the Cleveland Foundation grant, a CSU faculty members spent two summers developing the curriculum grid, working in concert with faculty responsible for the specific specialty courses to be certain community concepts and experiences were incorporated into the revised curriculum. This time line, however, enabled accomplishment off the goals within the targeted period.

Deterrents to all clinical experiences include unforeseen obstacles, false expectations, and communication breakdowns. Each of these factors contributed to some type of difficulty with the initial clinical experiences, but none was so serious that the project could not continue.

The formal program systems in the Cleveland neighborhoods are less structured than either the university faculty or the VNA staff. The programs have frequent staff turnover, rely on volunteers, and are subject to grant funding allocations and cycles. On occasion, communication was nonexistent, when, for example, a center would plan an activity in which students participation was desired outside the neighborhood but no coordination occurred with the faculty regarding days and times.

Students' Stereotypical Beliefs

A deterrent initially and until the program is long-standing are the stereotypical perceptions held by students of the neighborhoods and the people who live in the neighborhoods. These relate to non-familiarity with the setting and perceptions passed on from within the students' families, the student's neighborhoods, and prevailing social attitudes. Ongoing education removes the stereotypes, but initially causes students unnecessary stress and anxiety.

EVALUATION OF THE NEIGHBORHOOD-BASED CLINICAL EXPERIENCE

While benefits and deterrents were identified above, a formal system of evaluation of program effectiveness continues to be refined. Neighborhood systems continue to request services via Healthy Town nursing students' assignments, however, the effectiveness of services over time has not been determined.

The next logical step for the Vision project is to evaluate data that has already been gathered from the students and to refine our formal, longitudinal evaluation plan.

An additional expectation is to expand services to additional neighborhoods, based upon assessed community needs and projects responsive to those needs. Ongoing project needs are continued faculty development, development of additional sites, and Clinical Teaching Associates (CTAs) within those sites

We do know that, in the future, some measures of success of the Vision project will be:

- the number of graduates who are practicing in the community
- the evaluation of graduates' performances by employers
- the NCLEX pass rate now that students have less practice time in the acute care setting
- responses from graduates about their practice abilities

LESSONS LEARNED DURING THE DEVELOPMENTAL PROCESS

One of the major forces that contributed to the success of Vision on 22nd Street was the curriculum consultant. The Cleveland Foundation funded the consultant. This individual, a professor emeritus of education, had extensive experience with health care delivery systems. His role was facilitator, maintaining grant time lines, and objective observer. He maintained the integrity of the curriculum while addressing evaluation issues.

Group process and consensus-building techniques established trust among joint Vision faculty (CSU and VNA). A "shadowing" day for colleagues (VNA faculty) and academicians significantly increased respect for and knowledge about issues faced in each faculty's role. This "look into your world" bridged the gap voiced in joint discussions regarding roles and responsibilities in service delivery and academia.

The community faculty members and the VNA nurtured the partnerships in clinical education. Our multifaceted collaboration and networking facilitated access to neighborhood centers not previously available to the faculty. For example, the executive director of one center was highly enthusiastic toward the project and facilitated access to students in a variety of existing endeavors sponsored by the center including grant funded programs.

Obstacles Encountered

USE OF CLINICAL TEACHING ASSOCIATES (CTAS)

One unforeseen obstacle in the partnering with CTAs is the issue of their daily productivity requirement. Each VNA nurse is expected to make a certain number of visits per day. What would be the effect on that productivity if a RN student provided care for a patient from a CTAs caseload? How could the CTA be seen in respect to his or her peers? Problem resolution was that any patient followed by the student would still be counted in the daily productivity number for the CTA. The rationale was that the patient was still part of the CTA's workload and that the CTA spent time before and following the visit discussing the client and making sure all documentation was appropriate.

A second obstacle was the need to modify student's one day per week clinical schedule to be paired with certain CTAs. For example, if the CTA was a hospice nurse who worked only on certain days, then the student's schedule would need to change. For these situations, RN students who were able to flex their own work schedules were paired with hospice CTAs.

A similar obstacle with the CTA pairings arose when there was a vacation, illness, or leave of absence during a portion of the time when the RN student and the CTA were working together. These situations were addressed on an individual basis rather than reassigning the student to another CTA or rearranging the dates for student experiences so that the twosome could continue. An ultimate approach to overcome all of the above issues is to prepare more CTAs for teaching within the Vision model. It is hoped that some day all nurses within the VNA will be educated as CTAs.

EXPECTATIONS

Whenever discussions between a specific community center and faculty are initiated, directors, staff, and residents form expectations about the students' involvement. These expectations occur regardless of whether of not the discussions clearly identify the roles and expectations for the students or not. It is the responsibility of the faculty to carefully lay the groundwork, establish a process of open communication throughout the year, set guidelines for student participation in center activities, and then carefully attend to time commitments and the products of students' activities. The faculty must maintain close contact with center staff throughout the year to be certain that the expectations continue to be acceptable.

We have found that the longer the same faculty member is associated with a center, the greater the rapport, the fewer the obstacles, the more realistic the expectations, and the better the communication process.

COMMUNICATION

Communication issues related to the language of practice were found when CTAs became involved in the student's learning. Terminology used with the practice setting was found to differ from that being used by the faculty in the classroom. For example, what constitutes a home visit? What does it mean from the CTA's perspective and how does that differ from what the student has been taught? What protocols are automatically considered when terms like "home visit" are used? This situation has begun to be resolved through building a standardized vocabulary list with word or term definitions. Ongoing attention to differences in terminology and meaning is needed to prevent problems in this area.

A potential communication breakdown involves the complex information systems used by the VNA to assure quality service and maximum reimbursement. Special care is taken to be certain that students are knowledgeable with respect to documentation with the faculty taking the lead in orienting students and closely monitoring their client records.

DIFFERENCES OF CALENDAR

Working around the academic calendar, different university and community holidays and not being available in the summer has also created potential obstacles to be considered. With foresight, mutual development of expectations, and creative planning, this issue is dealt with on an ongoing basis.

SUMMARY

The creation of the Vision on 22nd Street model was driven by shared needs. The partnership has brought added value to each organization. Goals achieved include: a fully integrated, community-based curriculum; faculty enculturated in the concept of community-based care; students enculturation and preparation to practice in the community; and focused services to and maximization of existing health care and social service for Cleveland's urban neighborhoods.

REFERENCES

Antonovsky, A. (1979). *Health, Stress, and Coping*. San Francisco: Jossey-Bass.
Antonovsky, A. (1988). *Unraveling the Mystery of Health*. San Francisco: Jossey-Bass.
Benner, P. (1984). *From Novice to Expert*. Menlo Park, CA: Addison-Wesley.
Matteson, P. (1995). *Teaching Nursing in the Neighborhoods*. New York: Springer.
Selye, H. (1976). *The Stress of Life*. New York: McGraw-Hill.

10

A Violence Intervention and Prevention Program: The Experience of Northeastern University (Massachusetts)

Margaret A. Mahoney

Domestic violence is a serious public health problem. Latest estimates indicate that, each year in the United States, one million women and 1.4 million children are assaulted by a family member. Last year in Massachusetts, 22 men, women, and children were killed in domestic violence incidents (Boston Globe, Jan, 1998). Nationwide, 17% of all murder victims are killed by a family member, and more than 50% of all U.S. women who are murdered are victims of a current or former partner (Feldhaus, Koziol-McLaint & Amsbury, 1997). The prevention of violent and abusive behavior is a priority area in the national goals set by Healthy People 2000 (U.S. Department of Health and Human Services, 1997). It is imperative, then, that health care professionals are educated to screen and treat victims of violence appropriately. This chapter describes the joys and challenges that were experienced in our nursing program that provides community-based, interdisciplinary, experiential education in the area of violence prevention and intervention.

Northeastern University

Located in Boston, Massachusetts, Northeastern University is a private, urban institution that is student-centered and practice-oriented. The university encourages experiential learning by way of a cooperative education program through which students may alternate periods of traditional academic study with period of paid employment. The academic medical centers are within walking distance, and the nursing students often choose academic clinical placements and coop work placements as nurse's aides in these hospitals.

Involvement in the community has been a traditional practice at Northeastern. Because of its urban location, the university shares the concerns of traffic, crowding, pollution, and violence that seem endemic in large cities. Boston is a diverse city, with its population clustered in neighborhoods that are ethnically and culturally distinct. Northeastern's borders include the "Avenue of the Arts" to the north where Symphony Hall, the Museum of Fine Arts, Massachusetts College of Art, Wentworth Technological Institute, and Berklee College of Music can be found and the lower socioeconomic neighborhoods of Roxbury and the South End on the other two sides of the 55-acre campus. The latter neighborhoods have been designated by the federal government as being medically underserved.

Mission of the School of Nursing

In January 1999, the former College of Nursing became the School of Nursing, an organizational unit in the Bouvé College of Health Sciences. The mission of the School of Nursing is to provide "professional nursing education that prepares generalists . . . in nursing, contributes to the development of nursing science, provides service to the community, and advances the goals of the nursing profession" (NLN Self Study Report, 1991, p. 1). The faculty of the school defines the "focus of professional nursing practice as promoting, preserving, and restoring the health of individuals, families and communities. Professional nursing practice is an interactive process which promotes health and well-being and assists clients to adapt to a changing environment. The nature of nursing practice is independent, interdependent, and dependent, involving collaboration with health professionals" (NLN Self Study Report, 1997, p. 4).

The Faculty and Students of the Nursing School.

FACULTY

Thirty-five full-time faculty teach about 450 undergraduates and 350 graduate students. Additional part-time faculty are hired as needed for clinical instruction, and adjunct faculty are appointed to mentor faculty, precept graduate students, and enhance the education of the undergraduates. Many of the community faculty in the neighborhoods have been appointed to adjunct positions and contribute actively to the education of the nursing students. Because we employ a model that is community-based and interdisciplinary, many of the adjunct faculty are not nurses.

The faculty is organized in a unit structure that is based on the empowerment model of Wheeler and Chinn (1989). Operationalizing the core values of praxis, empowerment, awareness, consensus, and evolvement, the administrative structure is comprised of the Dean of the School, Assistant Dean for Administration, Directors of Graduate and Undergraduate Education, and Coordinators for Clinical Placement and Faculty Scholarship. Undergraduate course coordinators and graduate specialization coordinators also provide leadership in curriculum development, clinical placement selection, and evaluation.

STUDENTS

Because Northeastern is a private institution, tuition costs, educational preparation, and language are barriers to recruiting potential nurses from the residents of the neighborhoods that we serve. While we strive for diversity in the student body, the majority of the nursing students are from New England, with an average age of 23 years. The students are mostly Caucasian (86%), with some who are African American (7%), Hispanic (3%), Asian (3%), or Native American (1%). Seven percent of the student nurses are male (NLN Self Study, 1997, p. IV). The homogeneity of the student body makes the community-based, interdisciplinary education model an ideal vehicle for teaching cultural competence to these future nurses.

The Nursing Curriculum

In our community-based program, the students spend 50% of their clinical time providing health care to the residents of the inner city in collaboration with 10 neighborhoods. In an educational program that focuses on health promotion and disease prevention, they learn about the social, cultural, economic, and environmental factors that contribute to illness and disease. The rest of their clinical time is spent in acute, tertiary care facilities in the various nursing specialties. [Refer to Matteson, 1995 for further information.]

The nursing students begin their clinical education in the freshman year, with a skills lab that incorporates problem-based learning and computer-assisted instruction to enhance critical thinking skills along with psychomotor development for nursing care techniques. The introductory course includes process and skills, nursing history, care theories, professional issues, and ethics. In the sophomore year, the students begin their clinical experiences in a health promotion framework with a course on childbearing and child rearing followed by a course on health promotion through adulthood and old age. For both these courses, the clinical experiences are in the community, with healthy residents. The professional nursing role, health education, community assessment, communication, and cultural competence are emphasized. The upper-class students then move into the nursing specializations: pediatrics, mental health, acute care, and community. Their senior capstone course includes leadership, case management, and a precepted clinical experience that allows the student to gain skills in a specialty area of interest. (Refer to course list and sample program plan at end of chapter.)

Service Learning

Health professions education is moving some clinical learning experiences from an institution-based, highly technological approach to community-oriented partnerships and a health promotion approach. Students are also working with communities through service learning projects. The National Society for Experiential Education defines service learning as any carefully monitored service experience in which a student has intentional learning goals and reflects actively on what he or she is learning throughout the experience. Service learning programs emphasize the accomplishment of tasks which address community issues and include features which foster participants' learning about larger social issues and an understanding of the reciprocal learning and service which can occur between students and community members. (http://www.nsee.org) Based on this definition, community-based clinical education is not necessarily service learning. Service learning experiences, however, can be designed and incorporated into community-based nursing education.

James Joseph, in his keynote address to members of the Corporation for National Service (Fairfax, VA, 1994), identified three areas in the community: a public sector driven by ballot, a private sector driven by profit, and a volunteer sector driven by compassion. In order to prepare nurses to practice in the community, learning opportunities from each of these sectors are integrated into health profession education. The science and art of providing care to patients is now learned in the context of current policy concerning national health care initiatives, such as health maintenance organizations, and health care economics, such as the changes brought about by capitation. In this environment, special emphasis must be placed on students' having the opportunity to develop the compassion and empathy that are central to providing health care.

THE VIOLENCE INTERVENTION AND
PREVENTION (VIP) PROGRAM

When nursing students had the opportunity to work with survivors of violence, the lessons from each of the three community sectors (public, private, and volunteer) was brought into focus. Observing the political,
sociocultural, and economic forces that affect the care that is provided to
victims of violence had a profound impact on the professional development of the nursing students.

Overview of the VIP Program

The Violence Intervention and Prevention (VIP) program has been funded
for three years from the Health Professions Schools in Service to the Nation
Program, a national initiative of the Pew Charitable Trusts, the Corporation
for National Service, and the Bureau of Health Professions. The goals of
the HPSISN program are: to strengthen partnerships between health professions schools and communities which address unmet health needs; to
instill an ethic of community service and social responsibility in health professions schools, students, and faculty; and to equip the next generation of
health professionals with community-oriented competencies necessary to
practice in a changing health care environment.

The goals of this violence intervention and prevention program were
designed to operationalize the mission of the funding agency by focusing
on increasing awareness of relationship violence, teaching nurses to screen
all patients for violence and offering preventive services to the health centers and other community organizations. The clinical experiences were
designed on a service learning model, pairing student teams with Family
Advocates that were located in five health centers. Faculty development
sessions were held to educate the faculty about the impact of violence and
to develop curricula that would prepare the students and complement the
clinical experiences. Initial efforts with the students occurred through
directed studies and individual precepted experiences.

Synopsis of Educational Activity

Students first encounter the topic of domestic violence during the freshman year physical assessment course that includes screening for violence.
The topic of violence against women and children was introduced in the
first undergraduate clinical course. Elder abuse was taught in the adulthood and aging course. Mental health devoted a significant portion of the
curriculum to violence prevention in the community and the effects of vio-

lence in substance abuse and affective disorders. The acute care courses demonstrated the effects of family and street violence, with incidents of shaken baby syndrome and emergency room trauma. In the cultural diversity course, a violence seminar was conducted to address the special concerns of vulnerable populations: the undocumented, the disabled, the homeless, sex workers, and the lesbian population groups. In the community course, health policy and the social implications of our violent society were discussed.

Student clinical projects and research activities began to be focused on the impact of violence on population groups and individuals. Faculty research was initiated to develop and test innovative screening instruments and the influence on health care. A forensics course was developed as an elective for graduate students who wished to become more proficient in assessment of injuries, evidence collection and preservation, documentation, and providing expert testimony. Students who had taken an initial course were now asking for directed studies and coop experiences with family advocates or in hospital emergency rooms.

Neighborhood health centers adapted standards of practice and protocols across sites, and hospital emergency departments also hired advocates and developed "Jane Doe" admission policies. Faculty and students became politically active as members of the Governor's Task Force, the Massachusetts Nurses' Association Speakers Bureau, and the International Nurses' Network on Violence Against Women. A task force was appointed by the Provost to develop university guidelines to prevent violence on campus and to train a cadre of faculty to treat members of the Northeastern University community who are victims of violence.

Developing the VIP Program

The first objective of the VIP program was to strengthen existing partnerships and build new linkages between community-based organizations and health profession schools. Because we had been working in the neighborhoods with colleagues from the health centers, we utilized the existing networks established in the community to identify and arrange new collaborations.

Violence is a complex issue, and we needed to work across domains with primary care, mental health, social service, criminal justice, battered women's shelters, and victim witness advocates in the courts to develop our model of prevention and intervention. The students were placed in all of the above agencies for health promotion and service projects. Through their initiatives, providers of services learned about each other and organized formal workshops to plan interventions that spanned disciplines and traditional service areas. Representatives from these groups met monthly on an advisory committee to supervise the students and evaluate the program. Speakers were brought in to enhance skills and dialogue among service providers and faculty. Initial meetings were held at the university, then at each person's worksite so that all would gain a better appreciation for the environment in which advocacy for victims of violence occurs.

As the members of the advisory group strengthened existing relationships, new links were established through referrals and shared clients of concern. Pro bono lawyers were found, and the Northeastern law school students who are placed in emergency rooms for their clinical experiences became colleagues in identifying victims of violence. Another series of training sessions were held, incorporating the legal and medical perspectives.

Criteria for Selection of Neighborhood/Community Sites

Community sites for student learning experiences in violence prevention were selected from the 10 neighborhoods that had been providing clinical education to our students. Data from a community needs assessment conducted by the Center for Community Health Education Research and Service (CCHERS) indicated that the number one concern of residents in the neighborhoods was violence. Committed to trying to decrease the incidence of violence and develop the means to treat the victims of violence, the health centers chose to participate in this project. The five health centers that volunteered for this effort are located in Roxbury and Dorchester, areas of the city that have a high crime rate and are culturally diverse.

Based on the research, women are actually safer on the streets than in their own homes (Stuart & Campbell, 1989) where the risk of being murdered by a family member is four times greater (Campbell, Harris & Lee, 1995). In 1985, 45,011 women were murdered, 30% by a boyfriend or spouse (Stuart & Campbell, 1989). In 1991, the percentage of women killed by their partners rose to 50% (Campbell, Harris & Lee, 1995). Homicide is the leading cause of death of females aged 15 to 24 years, and a black female is four times more likely to be a homicide victim than a white female (Schnitzer & Runyan, 1995).

Although the fatality statistics are sobering, mortality data are easier to track than is the incidence of domestic violence which tends to be underreported. A 1985 national survey indicated that two million women, (16%) of all those who were married or cohabiting, were victims of violence. In 1991, six years later, this number had increased to 20% (Schnitzer & Runyan, 1995).

Of the 574,283 Boston residents recorded in the 1990 federal census, 10% live in Roxbury and 21% live in Dorchester. The racial breakdown is illustrated in the following table, by percent of the population:

	White	Black	Hispanic	Asian	Other
Boston	59.4	24.3	10.8	5.2	0.3
Roxbury	13.9	62.3	20.5	2.9	ns
Dorchester	31.6	48.5	15.4	4.0	0.5

Since the numbers of males to females is roughly equivalent in the population younger than 65 years, we can calculate that 20% of the females in the 15- to 64-year old category (with a 38% neighborhood average of two parent households) who might be at risk for violence is approximately 4,475 women. Neighborhood health centers that served this population were selected to be part of this violence prevention program.

Developing Clinical Leadership

There was much work done in advance to develop an infrastructure for the planning, coordination, and monitoring of the student activities in violence prevention and intervention. The VIP Program included funding for a student placement coordinator. Since no one would take this position for the amount of salary allocated in the grant, a partial salary was provided for two existing neighborhood health center coordinators who, in turn, agreed to work with the students for this project. The advisory team then chose to continue this model to obtain staff. Another grant was submitted to the Massachusetts Office of Victim Assistance, and support was obtained through federal funds under the Victims of Crime Act (VOCA) for coordinators in the three other neighborhood health centers. The VOCA grant enabled us to place our students with Family Advocates in five sites. In turn, the students are able to extend the capabilities of the Family Advocates.

The CCHERS neighborhood partners who were interested in the issue of violence prevention submitted a proposal to the Massachusetts Office of Victim Assistance (MOVA) to fund Family Advocates who would work 20 hours per week in five of the Neighborhood Health Centers. This grant was selected for funding July 26, 1995 through the federal VOCA funds (Victims of Crime Act) that are administered by the MOVA office which is governed by a Board chaired by the Attorney General.

The Family Advocates were hired from the neighborhoods, and each was a survivor of violence. There were intensive training sessions held so that the advocacy role could be learned and necessary resources and supervision established. Having a designated person who has expertise in the area of family violence in each clinical site gives more structure and accountability to the students' experience and makes a more formal link across health centers and between the health and criminal justice systems.

The Family Advocates expanded the health and social services currently available to victims by providing family advocacy and case management services specifically for adult and child victims of domestic violence. The Family Advocates provide direct services for identified victims of violence with social and legal advocacy, case management, client education, and consultation and training for provider teams, and they establish extensive linkages with the victim witness advocates in the courts and with other organizations providing services for identified victims of violence.

The family advocates serve as the preceptors for the HPSISN students who were placed in the health centers in groups, called Student Advocacy Teams. Since VOCA funds are designated solely for providing direct services to victims of violence, the students work with the Family Advocates to learn about intervention with victims of violence. In addition, the Student Advocacy Teams are responsible for providing the community education and prevention programs that the Family Advocates are not funded to do.

A Coordinating Team comprised of the leaders of the existing multidisciplinary Domestic Violence Task Forces at each site provides direction to the project and facilitates the sharing of resources and expertise across health centers. The members of the Coordinating Team also serve on the advisory committee to the HPSISN Violence Intervention and Prevention (VIP) Program. The Service Learning Coordinator for the VIP Program is also a member of the Coordinating Team, as is the Project Director and Project Evaluator from the college.

A training program was funded for the VIP Program faculty and was expanded to include the participants in the VOCA grant. The preparation and presentation of the VOCA proposal has served to strengthen our collaborative network and provides a clearer vision for the work of implementing a screening and intervention program in the neighborhoods. The projects are complementary, linking the educational goals of the VIP Program with the human resources needed to expand community services for domestic violence through VOCA.

Hurtles Encountered

PLACEMENT OF SERVICES

The health centers housed the advocate in their mental health units. This provided support systems for the advocates, but was a potential barrier to victims of violence who did not see themselves as having a "mental health" problem.

Another problem with the advocacy services within the mental health units was the issue of confidentiality. Not only did the students have a difficult time working with the victims directly, but also the primary care providers did not have access to the files or have communication about the interventions that were occurring. Victims were assured of confidentiality, often for very real safety concerns, which made the teaching/learning experience difficult.

SAFETY

The other concern was that the residents of the community all access the health centers for care. So, given the family-centered approach, the victims as well as the perpetrators were patients at the health center. Due to the close nature of these communities, violent incidents became well-known, and the staff at the health centers who live in the neighborhoods became concerned for their own safety.

Health centers, unlike hospitals, do not have security systems. Since they desire to be accessible to all, it was a real issue to provide services to victims of violence without compromising health care to other members of the family and community. The Boston police department was very helpful in providing safety assessments for the health centers and offering suggestions about emergency codes, alarm systems, and lighting in the parking lots. Training was offered to all staff, especially those at the front desk who felt most at risk when a victim's safety net was access to the health center.

CONCERN FOR STUDENTS

Initially, students often fear going into the inner city, for they hear about incidents of violence in the media. Orientation to the neighborhoods must include teaching about personal safety and "street smarts." Students are told not to wear expensive jewelry, carry money or purses, or walk alone at night. They are shown where to go in the neighborhoods if they need help and encouraged to get to know the local merchants and residents. As they become familiar with the neighborhoods, the students do not feel threatened by the environment. As they learn about the people and the community groups that enhance the quality of life in the neighborhoods, they are then in a position to develop interventions that are in concert with neighborhood goals and needs.

Violence can be shocking and needs to be introduced to the students in a clinical framework that enhances their understanding of their role as a professional nurse, not as a voyeur of the prurient side of life. The stories that the victims tell the students have brought tears to their eyes, but they become indignant when the victims tell of their treatment at the hands of professionals. The victims help to teach the next generation of nurses the mistakes not to make when working with their patients.

Safety concerns in the university setting were also discussed. If the statistic of 20% of women as potential victims is to be postulated then, in a typical nursing class in which violence is discussed, students will have personal experience with violence and some students will disclose to the faculty their history and fears. In order to prepare faculty to deal with this reality, training sessions were held, given by the Family Advocates, and a resource guide was compiled and distributed to each faculty member so that appropriate referrals could be made.

The Family Advocates in the neighborhoods came to include the university community in their scope of services, and sessions were offered about violence prevention and intervention yearly during Wellness Week on the Northeastern campus.

CONCERN FOR UNIVERSITY FACULTY

All faculty were given an inservice about the program and the curriculum during a faculty retreat. Participation in the program was through self-selection and curriculum reform. Even so, the program director served as an on-campus resource for faculty and taught in a variety of classes for the first two years of the grant. Guest lecturers were brought in from the community so that the students would have class content to support their community experiences.

During this process, the 20% statistic became evident. Because we are primarily a female faculty, this content struck a nerve with several faculty members who were now supported in sharing stories, long buried, with colleagues, Family Advocates, counselors, and, in some cases, students.

Disclosure does not happen without an environment of trust and support and assurance of confidentiality. Teaching about violence sensitizes the group to language and customs that promote its occurrence. For example, in preparing a Power Point presentation for a workshop on violence prevention, we decided to call the indentation markings "dots" instead of the usual "bullets."

CONCERN FOR THE FAMILY ADVOCATES

Relationships with the community partners began tenuously, but the goals of education and community service for health care professionals were difficult to achieve. The advocates were primarily survivors of violence and did not feel qualified to be in a Preceptor role. There was much support needed during the first year when they were funded for 20 hours a week and the students were an added responsibility. In the second year, their hours were increased to full-time and it was easier to accommodate the students, but their case loads were expanding rapidly, and, with the CDC grant coming at the end of the second year, the role demands became more complex. Many meetings were interfering with their ability to provide services to their clients which is their primary role. Balancing the needs of the community members with the needs of the students is the nature of this work, and other placements were sought for the third year.

Domestic violence work is challenging, and there are many job turnovers among the advocates and staff involved in the program. Working with survivors of violence has been a steep learning curve, and the physical, emotional, and psychological scars remain from that life experience. People who work with victims of violence need to be sure of a safe space for themselves—physical, emotional, and psychological. These accommodations needed to be made. When meeting one's basic living needs is a problem, there is no way one can add on another challenge like the education of health professions students. After three years, we are a lot more sensitive to the issues, but have learned by making mistakes.

Establishing trust is ongoing work—it is not given easily, nor is it sustained. The confidentiality and the privacy of the victims is closely guarded, for real safety reasons, but the students were not often given access to victims directly. There was real concern about victims being used by the students or "re-victimized" by unskilled novices in this arena. Students had to work with the advocates for a term before any access to survivors was granted. This process was repeated each cycle, and some students did not get past the gate-keeping activities.

Bridges Between Academia and Neighborhoods

The students who worked with the Family Advocates spent a portion of their clinical time engaged in a service learning curriculum model. They were placed in the health centers to provide service to victims of violence and to develop and implement activities that would prevent its occurrence. Service learning links curriculum goals with community needs so that no two clinical experiences are alike. The faculty worked closely with the neighborhood health center staff so that the student experiences could be well-planned. The students, however, could not expect to provide the "hand-on care" they often seek as preparation for being a nurse. The faculty were prepared to explain this other aspect of nursing care to students as well as the philosophy behind a service learning model.

Responsibilities of Students

Because of the issues of confidentiality and the need to establish trust, students were often not given access to victims until they had worked in the violence prevention program for several quarters. Many elected directed studies or coop experiences (funded through an AmeriCorps Higher Education Grant) to gain the continuity they needed to establish themselves as a member of the team, to participate in a support group, or to work in a battered women's shelter.

Responsibilities to the Neighborhood

Because of the trauma experienced by the victim of violence, we promised the neighborhood that we would not traumatize the victim again when she entered into care in the health center. Using patients to gain clinical experience by prying into their personal lives for our academic assignments, we may violate their trust and confidentiality. This fear is very real among advocates and survivors, and advocates were very protective of their clients.

Students and faculty were evaluated by the advocates and the survivors before trust and disclosure occurred. Students who wanted to participate in this program had to submit a resume and a cover letter stating their personal and professional experiences with violence and their goals for the experience. The family advocates reviewed these, and selected the students with whom they thought they could work. The projects for a term were discussed in the advisory group, and then negotiated with the students based on their time and their interest in the projects that were offered. Students often carried out their projects over several terms and sought to come back into the health centers during coops to complete their work or further develop their experiences.

RESULTS OF THE VIP NEIGHBORHOOD PARTNERSHIP

The focus of the Violence Intervention and Prevention (VIP) Program was to initiate domestic violence education for health profession students and provide community service for agencies working with victims of violence. Ten objectives formed the framework for the development and implementation of this project.

Review of the Objectives

FIRST OBJECTIVE

The first objective was to strengthen existing partnerships and build new linkages between community-based organizations and health profession schools. This objective has been met through the interface with the criminal justice system. Although there have been differing perspectives about working with victims of violence, the areas of intersection are much clearer in terms of role and the need to collaborate. It has been challenging to work with members of the criminal justice system, but the opportunity to understand each other's roles has enabled us to make more appropriate referrals.

SECOND OBJECTIVE

The second objective for the VIP program was to enhance awareness of family violence and service learning education among community providers. Through the family advocates, the health center staff have received training, clinical practice guidelines, and resource materials. They have come on campus to share their knowledge with other students. Student initiated research has helped to improve practice patterns and the reporting violence to providers in the health centers.

THIRD OBJECTIVE

The third objective was to provide family violence prevention services to the community through service learning projects developed and implemented by student advocacy teams. Multiple projects have been developed through the health centers, the schools, and the courts. The student teams were not as interdisciplinary as had been envisioned, however. The medical students were not often in the health centers at the same time as the nurse, and the course at BU had the service learning component as an option, not a requirement. The dental students were in their residencies and could not participate due to credit allocation and time constraints.

FOURTH OBJECTIVE

The fourth objective was to increase knowledge and skills in domestic violence for 25 health professional students in each year. This goal has been exceeded. There are between 20–25 students in each class at BU, and there have been three classes per year. The number of NU undergraduates range between 48–72 per class, and seven classes are taught each quarter. The graduate students average 10 per year per class, and 50% of them continue with their projects beyond the course through directed studies.

FIFTH OBJECTIVE

The fifth objective was to provide frequent opportunities for students to reflect on service learning experiences through an interdisciplinary seminar. This objective was more challenging. The first year, we scheduled seminars every other week at BU, and very few students from BU attended, although all of the Northeastern University nursing students were there. In the second year, we scheduled enrichment sessions with guest speakers once a month and had a fairly good response, but the numbers varied from 10 nursing students to 18 students from NU and BU together. Community members were also invited to attend these sessions, but few did. In the third year, we offered interdisciplinary training sessions and relied on the activities of the Dorchester Community Roundtable to bring folks together, which will be the ongoing mechanism for student involvement in interdisciplinary teams. In the third year, we also extended the program to another health center where all staff were trained.

SIXTH OBJECTIVE

The sixth objective was to establish an advisory group for the VIP program. This group was comprised of the family advocates from each health center, their supervisors, and the nursing faculty teaching the courses. During the first two years, this group met every month, did the planning and evaluation of the students' experiences, and organized the training sessions for the community sites. In the third year, with the CDC activities the meetings were cut to every other month. Participation went down, and there were more demands on the advocates' time. Their caseloads had built up, and they were more involved in direct service activities and less able to participate in this project.

SEVENTH OBJECTIVE

The seventh objective was to develop a program infrastructure for the planning, coordination, and monitoring of the service learning activities. In the grant, the positions of project evaluator and service learning coordinator were developed, but there was not enough money allotted in the budget to cover the demands of this role. There was turnover every year in this position, and the coordination fell to the project director. The evaluator was very helpful, but was also under-funded. The budget is one area in which lessons were learned that will impact planning for future grants. Since most of the grant money was allocated for training and health center expenses, there was not enough for faculty release time which would have been helpful as this project evolved. Providing funding for students was a positive step in that it encouraged their participation beyond the original course work.

EIGHTH OBJECTIVE

The eighth objective was to establish a program of university faculty development. Multiple training sessions were held, including a faculty retreat. A video library and resource material have been purchased to aid in teaching. Faculty development also occurred in the connections that were made in the community as a result of this program. Faculty practice is improved through knowledge of referral sources and informal networks of community support.

NINTH OBJECTIVE

The ninth objective was to integrate service learning and content on family violence into the core courses of the professional schools. This has been achieved in that domestic violence is integrated into the undergraduate and graduate curricula. Service learning and interdisciplinary community-based education has been fully integrated into the curriculum for the undergraduates and is beginning in the graduate program.

TENTH OBJECTIVE

The tenth objective was to sustain the VIP program beyond the end of the grant funding. Since the curriculum has been implemented at both schools, the educational initiative will continue. The community-based service learning opportunities will exist as the advocates have continued funding, and the need is great.

The materials produced as a result of this project include the protocols implemented at each health center that require all patients to be screened for domestic violence and the curricula at each participating educational institution that includes education about violence prevention and intervention for the health professions students. Other documents include the research projects that have been completed and are in the publication process.

EVALUATION

Evaluation of this project has been ongoing and process-oriented. The weekly student logs and reflection seminars have been the most helpful in terms of immediate feedback, and the advisory board meetings have helped to modify or redesign the service learning experiences. This was a transformational experience for the students in the program, and some of them have never left. Even after graduation, they continue with an active interest and professional participation in this area. They are bringing their knowledge and skills into their workplaces and applying the techniques that they have learned into their own practice settings. They are truly committed to this issue, and it has changed the direction of their lives. Many are actively involved with their own communities and politically active with professional organizations. They have offered to work with future students as well.

Other methods of data collection were through instruments developed for the Learn and Serve Project that tracked client contact, hours spent, and type of activity. These were less informative because the students filled them out sporadically, and many were incomplete. The students were required to spend 40 hours in the course, and this is the number they documented. The reality was that many spent much more time and richer information was obtained in the reflection groups.

The third instrument that was used for evaluation was the tool developed by the San Diego project. This instrument was used to evaluate the impact of service learning on the students. The responses indicated that the students were very satisfied that the service learning experiences were linked to classroom learning and enhanced the coursework. They were less satisfied with some of the actual community experiences. The impact on the community was more difficult for the students to assess, but they felt supported by the university in this project and were satisfied with the agencies.

When a survey was conducted in one health center to evaluate the impact of the training program, there were some very interesting results. Nearly one-third of the providers revealed that they had experienced violence in their own families and that this had an effect on their practice. Before the training sessions, 39% indicated that they felt well-prepared to intervene with victims of violence. After the training, this number increased to 69%. There were inconsistencies, however, with the protocol implementation, and only 70% of the providers screened all clients. The documentation of abuse and referral to social service went down after the training. A retrospective record review of patient charts in urgent care revealed that more men than women were screened for violence, a result of the urban street violence instead of family violence. This has implications for future training. The data also revealed that education alone does not produce behavior changes in screening patterns. There must be infrastructure and ongoing support services for intervention to occur. Without the infrastructure, providers may be less likely to screen, once they have been educated to all the complexities that domestic violence can present! This service learning project has been a transformational experience for the students and faculty. One staff member who received training disclosed that she had been in an abusive relationship and that the training had given her the knowledge and strength to end it. Several students have had this experience as well. This is an important point for faculty to consider who teach about violence. If one-third of the female population has been victimized, then one may expect to encounter survivors among colleagues and in classrooms. Having a working relationship with referral sources is important.

SUMMARY

One of the most important aspects of working with the VIP program is coming into personal contact with the statistics, with the conclusion that they are very real. The research data indicate that one out of three women encounter violence in their lives. The reality is that, in a female dominated profession such as nursing, the students and our colleagues are also victims of violence. We did not anticipate this as we began this program. As we talked about violence, we initiated disclosures among our colleagues and students that needed to be dealt with. We were not prepared for this, and it was very helpful to be connected with experts in the field who were willing to be referral sources. The provider surveys also supported the prevalence of violence among health care workers. Can we really expect them to intervene effectively when they may be in the same situation as the victim? This finding extends the theory of the cycle of violence into the workplace, an area of research that adds to the complexities of screening and intervention.

Part of the denial of the problem of violence in our society, apart from not seeing it in our peers, is that it is easier to screen clients who differ from us by race, class, socioeconomic, gender, religious preference, culture, or sexual preference. Victims will seek a safety zone, for physical, psychological, and emotional safety. Providers will do the same. Advocacy skills need to be taught, and practice opportunities need to be created safely in clinical settings.

What we also discovered from the research was that education alone does not mean that providers will screen for violence. Less than 50% of the patients who presented at the clinic with injuries were screened for domestic violence. Out of the patients who were screened, 52% were male. The conclusion that we could draw from this is that, while we were educating providers about relationship violence, the clients who were walking into the clinic were victims of urban violence. We need to tailor our approaches to meet the needs of the patients that the clinicians are actually seeing.

Another barrier to providing academic education in the area of domestic violence is that there is a lack of a theoretical base for the screening activities. We are hypothesizing, based on the data from the evaluation project, that the theory of Silencing the Self (Jack, 1993) may be applicable to this population. A future project will be to conduct key informant interviews to link the provider's experiences to the concepts in the model as the basis for a future study of the variables that affect screening patterns in the providers.

Working with victims also allows and encourages us to identify patterns of victimization in our colleagues and students. The "victim mentality" has sensitized us to the power differentials that exist in the field and to the need to exercise caution in using this power inappropriately. This is one example of transformational experiences leading to changed priorities, community activism, and political engagement in this arena. The feminist notion of "giving voice" to the problems of domestic violence has required courage to engage in an area that the majority of the population prefers to keep hidden.

Collaborating with other disciplines, we became aware of how our perspectives and work view shapes our perceptions and values. Where we sit determines where we stand on the issues that are important to us. The power and control that come into play when working on collaborative research projects and how we demonstrate respect for students, victims, members of other disciplines, and neighborhood residents have been amply demonstrated in the conduct of this project. The importance of ethical practice and the deep-seated needs of the victims of violence and the residents of the neighborhoods have been motivating factors for the faculty and students involved in the VIP program. In the words of Socrates, "It is better to suffer evil than commit it, because the former only harms my body, but the latter corrupts my soul." This helps to find the courage to confront the problems inherent in working with victims of violence in the neighborhoods, and to not be silent on their behalf.

REFERENCES

Campbell, J., Harris, M. & Lee, R. (1995). *Violence research: An overview. Scholarly Inquiry for Nursing Practice: An International Journal, 9*(2), 105–126.

College of Nursing. (1997). *Northeastern University College of Nursing Self Study Report*, Boston, MA: Author.

Fullilove, M. (1996). *Patterns of violence*. In Filtcraft, A., Pilchta, S., Mazure, C. M., Bunney, B. S. & Scott Collins, K. (Eds) *Violence against women in the United States: A comprehensive background paper.* (2nd ed.) pp. 7–25, NY: Commonwealth Fund Commission on Women's Health.

Greenfield, L. (1998). *Violence by intimates: Analysis of data on crimes by current or former spouses, boyfriends, and girlfriends.* Washington, D.C.: U.S. Department of Justice.

Jack, D. C. (1993). *Silencing the self: Women and depression.* New York: Harper.

Matteson, P. (1995). *Nursing Education in the Neighborhoods: The Northeastern University Model.* New York: Springer.

Office of Research and Health Statistics (1994). *Neighborhood Health Status Report: The Health of Dorchester*, Division of Public Health, Trustees of Health and Hospitals, Inc. City of Boston.

Schnitzer, P. & Runyan, C. (1995). *Injuries to women in the United States: An overview. Women & Health, 23*(1), 9–27.

Stuart, E. & Campbell, J. (1989). *Assessment of patterns of dangerousness with battered women. Issues in Mental Health Nursing, 10*, 245–260.

United States Department of Health and Human Services. (1990). *Health People, 2000: National health promotion and sidease prevention objectives.* Washington, D.C.: Author.

Wheeler, C. E., & Chinn, P. L. (1989). *Peace and power: A handbook of feminist process.* (2nd ed.). New York: National League for Nursing.

11

Educating Nursing Students in the Neighborhoods: Lessons Learned

Peggy S. Matteson and Eileen Zungolo

A community-based pedagogy provides a substantive and stimulating component to the education of future nurses. It encourages those involved to develop an understanding of the interconnecting relationship among ideology, power, and culture. Students learn how to provide care from the people of the community, no matter where they are or their level of health care needs. The three constituents—members of the university, providers in the community, and members of the community—work together to create and implement the program of services. By responding to the needs identified by community members, each neighborhood provides a unique context for education.

The programs described in the prior chapters showcase the diverse ways in which community-based education may be implemented. Incorporating the key elements of: (1) true partnership, (2) community voice, (3) services emerging from the capacities of the community and nursing program and (4) interventions responding to needs identified by the neighborhoods served, each school has developed a unique program.

Establishing and maintaining a community-based clinical program requires us to expand our view of the process of nursing education while simultaneously developing new teaching approaches and skills. Change like this is not a smooth or easy process. We have noted, however, 10 prevalent lessons that will facilitate your development of a successful community-based nursing education program.

LESSON 1
KNOW YOUR CULTURE

As nurse educators, we reside simultaneously in multiple cultures, two of which are the culture of education and the culture of nursing. In our work we are constantly bridging the span between education and practice, explaining to our colleagues in education the dimensions of a program of clinical education while simultaneously explaining to our colleagues in practice the educational requirements our students must achieve. We function as conduits between these two cultures. With community-based nursing education, we are interacting with additional cultures. We must now interpret the cultures of nursing and education to our community partners.

In exchange, they will instruct us about their culture(s). To understand why someone behaves as she does you must understand how the situation looked to her, what she thought she had to contend with, and what alternatives she saw open to her. This is true not only for us to understand our clients needs and actions but also for our clients to understand our needs and actions.

LESSON 2
RESPECT THE OWNERSHIP OF THE COMMUNITY.

Each neighborhood belongs to the people who reside there. We enter as guests and can only understand the affects of opportunity structures, social norms, and other commonly evoked explanations of human behavior by seeing them from the resident's point of view. We may hear from the leaders, but we must also learn from the individual residents. Each individual offers his or her own perspective; collectively, they provide a composite view of their realities.

We enter a neighborhood at a specific point in its development. Learn the history of the area. The growth of a neighborhood and its people offers you important background information. The events of the past will not only influence your reception, but also the future development of your partnership.

LESSON 3
INVITE DIVERSITY

To develop and support the diversity of the partnership, it must be constantly inclusive while steadily building consensus. Consensus brings together the diverse efforts and resources creating the power for change. Seek out potential partners in facilities and neighborhoods that represent heterogeneity. Connect with the underserved, disenfranchised, or disempowered. Honor their uniqueness. Whether they are disassociated due to apprehension, lack of money, transportation, employment or insurance, language or cultural isolation, or mental or physical disabilities, these are people with the capacities for partnership. As they come to trust you and gradually let you into their world, you will met some very strong, very resourceful people. Their health concerns and ability to respond to health services will engage students and put them in touch with the reality of peoples' lives

LESSON 4
BUILD THE VISION TOGETHER

As the partnership develops, all participants provide input into the development of the vision. Participating in the dialogue enables participants to achieve significance and develop mutual trust as they collaborate in the development of their vision.

A vision provides direction. A united vision is vital for cohesiveness. With an articulated vision the steps to achieving it can then be identified, and ownership for various tasks may be accepted. A vision without tasks remains a dream, tasks without a vision providing purpose is drudgery. But when we combine a vision with tasks we can make a difference.

LESSON 5
THE HEART IS MORE IMPORTANT
THAN THE HEAD

We come to the neighborhood offering both our services and ourselves. In order to develop a partnership, we must become emotionally involved in their joys and concerns, and we must learn about and value, what is important to them. This knowledge provides the ability to empathize, to see things from their perspective. Without this connection, we will miss important aspects of their defenses against threats, their reactions to crises and problems, and the limits of their tolerance. If we don't offer what is in our hearts, what is in ours heads won't matter.

LESSON 6
BEING IS MORE IMPORTANT THAN DOING

This lesson follows closely on the concept of leading with the heart. Being with someone incorporates the idea of mutuality, of joining with someone where they are, of being available to them. Sitting and having a cup of coffee or sharing a meal honors the other by demonstrating a regard for them through the everyday ritual of taking refreshment together. Through this process we connect with others as valued human beings, someone to do things with collaboratively.

This present of presence becomes the platform on which the partnership is built and the caring relationships develop. Faculty can model for students how to engage others in such a manner, how to listen, and more importantly, how to respond to what is being shared.

LESSON 7
DEVELOPING A GENUINE PARTNERSHIP TAKES TIME.

Remain patient. Partnerships can only be built on trust, and building trust takes time. In the past, neighborhoods have been used to further the educational and research agendas of others. The community gatekeepers have become cautious because these past intrusions from academia have not been useful to the residents. The word "Tuskeegee" is widely known among minority groups and they are hesitant to be victimized again.

To be authentic partners, we must engage in developing reciprocal agreements with each neighborhood. These will outline the reality we will mutually seek to transform and the way in which this will be done. This is the first step in the process of partnership development. Once committed, we must be reliable in our efforts, be faithful in our interactions, and finish what we start. Success will lead to an increased amount of trust that will, in turn, lead to more opportunity within the partnership.

Community-Based Nursing Education

LESSON 8
WELCOME CREATIVE CONFLICT

All will not flow smoothly! This pedagogy brings together multiple cultures, speaking from different perspectives without a common language. (Even the cultures of nursing academia and nursing practice speak different languages.) In addition, each constituency has a different agenda. Each group speaks from different experiences. There will be a difference of opinion as to what is to be done, how it will be done, and the prioritizing of when it will be done.

Don't be discouraged when there is disagreement. Actually, verbalization of disagreement is good. It means the participants trust each other enough to risk dissention and disagreement. The best part is that when you know what people are thinking, you know where the work needs to be done to further develop the partnership.

A partnership is a planned, long-term association with a convergence of goals. It is based on a perception of greater strength and possibility of success by working together and is pulled forward by a mutual vision. Partnerships, however, move in an optimistic uncertainty. It is this combination that encourages creativity.

LESSON 9
IT'S ABOUT PROGRESS, NOT PERFECTION

Each neighborhood partnership begins with ambiguity. Embrace that state as it means that very little is pre-determined. You have room for joint creativity. Start by working in the present with small ventures while constantly looking and building towards the future. Every interaction, every activity facilitates the next one. When you know better, you will do better (Maya Angelou).

LESSON 10
DOING TOGETHER IS MORE IMPORTANT
THAN DOING ALONE

We are creating a neighborhood-based educational partnership. The process demands that there be ongoing, collaborative efforts between faculty, students, neighborhood providers, and neighborhood residents. We must explore, dialogue, eat, plan, play, take risks, laugh, and celebrate together. Success will occur when we learn from our partners, work from mutually developed objectives, negotiate our roles, and fulfill our promises!

INDEX

Ⓢ *Springer Publishing Company*

Distance Education in Nursing
Jeanne Novotny, PhD, RN

Pioneers of Internet-Based education programs in nursing schools around the country share their expertise in this "how to" guide for the design and implementation of distance education. Includes contributions from the nurses at the University of Colorado, University of Phoenix, the Frontier School of Midwifery, and Vanderbilt University. For nurse educators of undergraduate, graduate, advanced practice and RN students.

Contents:
- Introduction
- Distance Education Foundations
- Teaching a Web-Based Course: Lessons From the Front
- Software Tools for Web-Based Course Development
- Clinical Applications of Electronic Learning Systems
- Focus on the Learner
- Assessing Distance Education Programs in Nursing
- Promoting Informatics in the Nursing Curriculum
- Distance Education at the University of Phoenix
- Distance Graduate Education: The University of Colorado Experience
- Nurse Practitioner Education: The Virginia Experience
- Distance Education at the Frontier School of Midwifery and Family Nursing: From Midwives on Horseback to Midwives on the Web
- Supervision of RN Distance Learning Students: The Experience of Vanderbilt's RN Bridge Program
- A Model for Development of a Web-based Trauma Course
- An International Education Model: The Experience of the School of Nursing at the Catholic University of Chile
- The Future of Nursing Education: Marketability, Flexibility, and Innovation

2000   280pp.   0-8261-1341-9   hard   www.springerpub.com

536 Broadway, New York, NY 10012-3955 • (212) 431-4370 • Fax (212) 941-7842

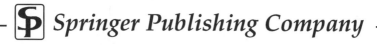

Springer Publishing Company

American Nursing
A Biographical Dictionary, Volume 3

Vern L. Bullough, RN, PhD and **Lilli Sentz,** Editors

Sharon Richardson, Bonnie Bullough, Olga Church,
Contributing Editors

"As far as I know, none of this type of material is yet online in any of the databases related to nursing history."

—Joan Lynaugh
Center for the Study of the History of Nursing
University of Pennsylvania School of Nursing

This exciting collection traces the development of the nursing profession through the biographies of individual nurses since 1925. The list of several hundred names, compiled through the help of nurse historians and volunteers from the American Association for the History of Nursing, features notable nurses Faye Abdellah, Virginia Henderson, Margaret Kerr, and Thelma Schorr. It gives nurses a real sense of their history which is not available anywhere else. The contributors of the biographies in an act of scholarly devotion preserve a sense of the profession's past.

American Nursing: A Biographical Dictionary, Volume Three is an invaluable reference work for students and librarians. Fully illustrated with many one-of-a-kind photographs.

2000   328pp.   0-8261-1296-X hard   *www.springerpub.com*

536 Broadway, New York, NY 10012-3955 • (212) 431-4370 • Fax (212) 941-7842

JACKSON LIBRARY - LANDER UNIV.

3 6289 00269159 7

DATE DUE

DEMCO 38-297